Mini Habits for Fitness

Fitness

The 60-Day Plan to Rebuild Your Relationship with Exercise

By
Stephen Guise

minihabits.com

Copyright & Disclaimer

Contents

Introduction

Important Definitions and Ideas

Habit: a behavior performed so often that your subconscious mind learns to prefer it and may even do it thoughtlessly. A habit means less thought and effort go into the behavior. If it isn't a decision, it's a habit.

Mini habit: a "stupid small" behavior that you complete every day (see next page for examples). These are completely functional, smaller-than-usual habits and the perfect foundation for learning to love a behavior.

Stupid small: a challenge so small and easy that it sounds stupid. You'll laugh at it. You'll scoff at it. That's why you'll be able to crush it every day.

Bonus reps: extra repetitions beyond your initial mini habit. These are encouraged, but optional.

Mini Habit Exercise List

There are a couple of ways to go about this. I started my mini habit over a decade ago with one push-up per day. If you want variety, however, you can simply choose an option from this list each day. Or you can simplify your daily goal by saying 60 seconds of any type of intentional exercise each day.

If you make your mini habit one minute minimum and you feel any resistance, make it even smaller (30 seconds is a great place to start). Don't choose 10 minutes, even though it sounds easy. Having a 100% success rate is critical to your success with this strategy, and, on your worst days, 10 minutes of something you don't want to do is a bigger ask than you might think.

Choosing 10 minutes seems bolder than one minute, but it's

actually playing scared. It means you're afraid that one minute isn't enough. It means you're afraid that you won't or can't do bonus reps unless you aim for them initially. Both are patently false and proven wrong by hundreds of thousands of people (myself included). The initial mini target serves three purposes:

1. Too small to fail. You can do it on your worst day.
2. Short-term momentum: leverage this small win into a bigger win (bonus reps).
3. Long-term momentum: every day you win builds strength in the behavior, ultimately changing your relationship with exercise.

Here are some mini habit ideas.

Mini Habits by Quantity

- 1 push-up
- 1 sit-up
- 1 pull-up
- 1 yoga pose
- Run up and down the stairs twice
- Walk or jog to the end of your driveway, block, or mailbox
- Walk an extra 1,000 intentional steps (or set a step target a bit more than your average, but not 10,000 steps, which is too much for our strategy and not a scientifically relevant number)

Mini Habits by Time (30 sec recommended for beginners)

- Run (outside, treadmill, stairs, in place)
- Walk
- Plank

- Dance (for 30 seconds or to one song)
- Jumping jacks
- Push-ups
- Sit-ups
- Pull-ups
- Miscellaneous exercise(s)

Other Options
- Start an active video game such as *Thrill of the Fight* or *Beat Saber* and play as long as you want
- Put on your gym clothes (I'm serious. Don't underestimate this one.)
- Set up your exercise mat, press play on a workout video, sit on the mat (you don't have to do the workout, but make yourself do this much and you'll probably want to do at least a little bit, right?)

Final public service announcement: 10 or 20 minutes is not a mini habit for most people. Five minutes could be a mini habit for some people, but is not recommended to start with. Make your behavior so easy you can't ever say no! That means you will still do it when you forget about it all day, are dead tired, and need to go to bed in the next five minutes. I've done my push-up mini habit in my bed before. Easy wins and long winning streaks are the power behind this idea!

Start Right Now

Before we get any further into the book, start your mini habit right now.

We won't start counting for real until you reach Day 1, but your mini habit is so small and easy that you can "practice" every day until then. Simply choose a habit from the provided list (or create your own) and commit to doing it once every day before you go to sleep. If you're a planner, set a specific time each day. If you're a spontaneous person like me, just get it done at some point. If you realize you're about to sleep and haven't done it, do your mini habit right then and there before your head hits the pillow.

You always have the option to do "bonus reps" whenever you feel extra motivation toward your fitness goals. Or you can stop at the minimum and declare it a win--that's completely fine!

After the introduction, I will explain the detailed plan for our 60 days. Following that, Day 1 officially begins.

Depending on how much and how fast you read, today might be Day 1, or it might be Day Negative 4. It's totally up to you! The reason I encourage this early start is that it is mentally healthy to learn to do your mini habit (and exercise in general) without getting "official credit" for it.

Social media and fitness trackers can often turn exercise into something we check off a list or do for external validation like likes or clout. These aren't inherently bad as supplemental motivation sources, but they are not indicative of a fully healthy and self-sustaining relationship with exercise.

We want to get to a point where we view exercise the way we view tacos. We want tacos and pursue tacos for the sake of tacos, not because of any external pressure or motivation.

Why This Book?

I've written *Mini Habits*. I've written *Elastic Habits*. I've written *Mini Habits for Weight Loss*. So why write *Mini Habits for Fitness*?

This book's unique format will offer something different from all of the above. This is a daily guide where you read just a 1-2-page section each day of your fitness habit journey. By focusing on fitness, I can tailor the best behavior change strategy to the world's most desired habit.

It's one thing to exercise. It's another to change your relationship with exercise. Many aspiring exercisers see it as a necessary evil. What if you saw your marriage like that? Perhaps some do, but I think we can agree that "necessary evil" is not the foundation you want for a healthy relationship.

The "perfect" marriage would have love and respect and enjoyment of each other's company. The same goes for the perfect relationship with exercise. Gym rats, fitness freaks, weightlifting wasps, and yoga yaks tend to have one thing in common--they love to exercise. They don't merely love the results of exercise. They love the entire process.

Why do you think some people are addicted to exercise while others have to fight themselves to work out?

That's simple. It's based on each person's relationship with physical activity.

The key to getting fit isn't a $4,000 treadmill. That would be like saying the key to a healthy marriage is to find the right house. Sure, a nice treadmill that fits your lifestyle can enhance your experience, just as a nicer house may introduce fewer problems than an old house, but the core determinant of success and failure is the relationship quality itself. Wealthy couples in mansions split up all the time despite having access to everything money can buy, while poor couples develop an unbreakable bond. Nice home gyms may go unused as those with fewer resources use sandbags and jugs of water as weights every day.

Fitness is never determined by access to equipment or location, as we can exercise with nothing but our own bodyweight.

If you want to get fit, then your best bet is to learn to love physical activity. I've personally gone from hating working out to loving it because of a mini habit, and, trust me, this is a fun change from the normal approach.

My books have worked so well for myself and others in part because I'm an ideal guinea pig. To be blunt, I'm lazier than most people. I'm not driven by routine, which is a huge disadvantage for habit development. I want to play all day. Being productive is not easy for me. I desire to live well despite my hedonistic inclinations.

I don't know about you, but I've tried the hard way. It didn't work. And why should that surprise me? I prefer the easy way. I don't have the work ethic of Kobe Bryant or the determination of David Goggins. Just because you see and understand and are inspired by someone like David Goggins does not mean you can imitate it well (or at all). My limitations have forced me to find creative strategies to get myself to work, exercise, and so on.

Most strategies require you to be a super version of yourself each day, and that's why they fail.

This strategy allows you to be yourself and live your life as usual. Even the busiest, laziest, and tiredest person can add a simple mini habit to their day; you will be amazed as it changes you from the inside out. We don't get to become super versions of ourselves by wanting it; we get there by training to become it.

Your Relationship with Exercise

I'd rather make a spreadsheet than wrestle a bear, but I'll admit the latter is more exciting and a better workout. Alas, modern life has changed our default relationship with exercise (more spreadsheets and less bear wrestling). Exercise was once a necessary part of living--bear hunting and all--but now it's possible (and in many ways encouraged) to live with limited movement.

Look at me right now. I'm writing on a laptop on my couch. It's 71 degrees Fahrenheit in my house. Between my lap and the laptop is a soft throw blanket. From this same couch, I can order food to be delivered to my door just a few feet away. I could practically live on this couch! And while I feel like I want to do that, I really don't want to do that, because sedentary living comes at a high cost.

Right now, it would be easy to point out the scary "sitting" statistics. YOU WILL DIE IF YOU SIT ON THE COUCH TOO LONG. DOOOOOM! Blah blah. Shame shame shame. That's not what anyone needs.

While it's true that sedentary living has morbid studies and statistics about it, a threat-based approach is foolish because it can easily *worsen the problem*! Why? It worsens our relationship with exercise.

Who has ever fallen in love with something or someone because they were threatened by it or by someone in relation to it? Maybe it has happened (shotgun weddings), but that's no path to a lasting bond.

Now think about this. How often have you approached exercise from an angle of wanting results, a sense of obligation, or to ward off the threat of poor health? I'm guilty of it. It's understandable why we'd drift into this mindset, but since we can see this is not exactly a fun mindset, is it necessary for results? Is it optimal to threaten and shame ourselves into taking more walks?

Step Back and See the Simplicity

Exercise is simply movement. It's natural, like eating. We don't feel obligated to eat; we eat because it's life-sustaining, it benefits us, and it's fun.

But Stephen, eating is way more fun and even more necessary than exercise. I agree, but they are much closer than they seem. Exercise is not defined as a grueling and sweaty hour in the gym, it's merely movement in all of its forms, and we all move every day. Thus, we all readily exercise every day already. And we need to move to carry out various tasks. When it comes to exercise, it's strictly a matter of dosage, then. You probably bought this book because you think it'd benefit you to move more.

Recognizing this simple fact is a big deal because it takes you away from the all-or-nothing mindset that keeps people sedentary. You move every day, even without trying to "exercise." Don't perceive this as "doing nothing." Your mini habit is the intentional exercise seed that will naturally expand your repertoire of natural daily movements.

Daily Movement has Changed

When Caveman Mack speared a deer, he did it to survive. He didn't return to the cave and say to his family, "Hey, fam, I got 10,000 steps and venison today." The movement he needed to achieve his goal was an afterthought, yet that movement gave him great benefits.

Movement to humans was once no different than eating,

drinking, or breathing; it was natural, expected, and, in that way, effortless. Modern technology has eliminated significant naturally required movement from the modern lifestyle in the name of convenience. But, as they say, "nothing is free."

We've lost the natural movement that once made physical activity effortless. When things come naturally to you, you don't perceive them as requiring much effort (even if they require a lot of it). The scientific terminology for this phenomenon is perceived effort. I wrote about this in the original *Mini Habits* book. Perceived effort is a big cog in the habit formation system because the same behavior...

1. can feel different to two different people
2. can feel different to the *same person* in the same moment (depending on their mental approach/mindset)
3. can feel different to the same person over time (as the relationship changes)

I was born Stephen Guise, and let me check... yep, I'm still him. Same genetics and everything. But I'm a materially different person than I was 15 years ago. I've changed. Today, going to the gym for one hour feels fun and rewarding. Fifteen years ago, it felt daunting and monumental. Same person, different perception of effort.

Briefly, let me describe day one, the day that ultimately birthed the *Mini Habits* idea. I was too intimidated/lazy/depressed/sluglike to do the 30-minute workout I felt I "should" do. The perceived effort of this workout exceeded my ability. But thanks to a creative thinking book called *Thinkertoys*, I thought about doing the opposite of an intimidating workout. One push-up!

When I did that one push-up, I created momentum, and that helped me do another, and another. Then, 30 minutes later, I had completed the aforementioned "impossible" 30-minute workout.

It was the same thing I couldn't do before.

My perceived effort started sky high, but I figured out how to lower it and won.

Perceived effort explains why I can play basketball for three hours straight (fun) but look at my watch after 10 minutes on the treadmill (working out for a result). I'll burn more calories playing basketball, but it feels easier. And with that, we've peeled back a major layer of this puzzle-onion.

Technology has reduced our natural movement. Many of the chores that are unnecessary now with technology once brought us great movement benefits. Washing clothes used to entail lots of scrubbing and beating clothes on rocks.

For most of human history, exercise was a natural and secondary effect of living. Today, it feels more like a separate chore we "should" do: high pressure, judgment-filled, and mechanical. This skyrockets the perceived effort and difficulty of exercise. We must rediscover it as close to its original form as possible.

This same thing happened to me as a boy, but with reading. I loved reading *Goosebumps* and *Choose Your Own Adventure* books. It was fun. Then, I started getting homework at school. Suddenly, I was required to read. Uh-oh.

You might think that required reading shouldn't be a problem since I naturally enjoyed reading, but the relationship changed when I couldn't choose my reading content, when I read, or how much I read. Reading went from free and exploratory to restrictive and forced. It went from "I love reading" to someone telling me "You must read." This sounds a whole lot like what happened to the human race with physical movement, doesn't it?

As the years went on, I grew to despise reading (which I once loved). Looking back, there never was anything about reading itself that I despised. My relationship with reading was spoiled by pressure to read. Not everyone responds this way to reading homework, I know. But I did and I don't think I'm the only one.

There are billions of people whose relationship with exercise has been strained or spoiled in exactly this way. And that's a shame, because exercise can be everyone's greatest ally. What's more satisfying than using your body's gift of movement, making it stronger, and reaping the most incredible benefits of any behavior in the world?

The Real Benefits of Fitness

You may debate me on this, but the best reason to exercise is not external. It's not six-packs, bulging muscles, slim waists, and sexy bodies. *It's internal.* I know everyone wants to look better. But physical appearance can't compare to the internal transformation of someone as they get fitter.

The suite of internal benefits of being fit is immense: mental clarity, increased energy, a general sense of well-being, confidence, and having a body that can weather sickness or other physical challenges. Health is wealth, as they say, and fitness is the primary pathway to better health.

Exercise is like *magic inside the body.* The reason gym rats exist is because exercise is addictive, internally and externally. If you're going to be addicted to something, I can't think of a better choice.[1]

Here's a quote from a well-known exercise addict:

"The greatest feeling you can get in a gym, or the most satisfying feeling you can get in the gym is... The Pump. Let's say you train your biceps. Blood is rushing into your muscles and that's what we call The Pump."

~ Arnold Schwarzenegger

Here's the greatest bodybuilder of all time, talking about a benefit that you can feel your *first* time lifting weights. "The Pump" is an ancillary (not primary) benefit of exercise, but these kinds of benefits are important and satisfying too. You feel stronger after lifting weights because of "The Pump." You temporarily look stronger because of "The Pump." Eventually, The Pump fades, but it's like a sneak preview of what you'll look like if you keep lifting weights.

We'll talk more about the benefits of exercise throughout our 60-day journey. I'll share my favorite quote about what exercise does for us on Day 24. It's one of the things that helped me "get" exercise, and why it benefits so many health and wellness markers. Don't skip ahead and read it yet. On Day 24, when you read it, you will understand it fully because of your experiences leading up to it!

Daily Format

This is a daily guide for a reason. Over 10 years and five books later, I've taken note of the three biggest challenges people have faced when building mini habits.

Mini Habits Challenges
1. People think these behaviors are too small to matter (or believe they are inferior to larger ones).
2. People give up before their habits form.
3. People struggle to detach from typical goal psychology.

To address these challenges, in this book, I'm not merely describing a system for building your fitness habit that you have to remember forever. Instead, I'm going to *show you*, every step of the way. Day 5 is going to be written differently than Day 49, because those are wildly different phases of the journey.

I've studied human behavior and habit formation for more than 15 years. I know the general process of habit formation. **Thus, I can give you information near the time you'll need to hear it. I can predict...**

- when you'll face the most resistance.
- when you need a reminder of the process and reasoning behind it.
- when the behavior begins to transition from conscious to subconscious.
- when you'll wonder if small habits are enough.

I won't get the timing perfectly correct, of course, as habit formation isn't 100% orderly and linear (and varies by behavior and person). But I can get close enough to warn you of something that will happen soon or explain something that has just happened.

This format aims to improve your understanding of the whole process and help you see exercise in a new way.

I'm confident this will be the most effective fitness book you've ever read. Stick with this for 60 days, and you'll be well on your way to a powerful fitness habit to improve your health, physique, strength, mind, and ability for the rest of your life.

After reading a book, it only stays with you as long as you remember it or revisit it. Unless you reread the same book multiple times, a strong memory and mindfulness are required for success. In essence, books struggle to hold people accountable and support them *after* being read. We will change that dynamic right now.

Daily Format Benefits:
- The easy daily read serves as a trigger for your mini habit (build a reading and exercise habit simultaneously!).
- Information is delivered in a timely and relevant manner instead of in one big chunk that you need to remember and recall for months.
- 60 days should be enough time to develop a habitual foundation with an easy mini habit.

You can expect some repetition. This is by design! Repetition improves retention of concepts, as well as familiarity and acceptance of concepts.

Repetition improves retention of concepts.

Repetition improves retention of concepts.

Repetition improves retention of concepts.

Most exercise programs only focus on your behavior. Do this. Do that. We're aiming to improve your thought patterns and perception of exercise as we help form your behavior with daily repetition. Daily repetition combined with thought training will move the needle twice as fast in theory. But how can we test that theory? I'm glad you asked!

Let's begin by seeing where you are now.

Assessment Quiz

Exercise is movement: walking, jogging, running, lifting

weights, dancing, bodyweight exercises, stretching, yoga, playing sports, and so on. Each person has a unique relationship with individual types of exercise, a broader relationship with general movement, and a relationship with different intensities of movement.

Example:

✓ Jennifer hates hockey because it knocked her teeth out. (Individual)
✓ Jennifer loves yoga because it feels great. (Individual)
✓ Jennifer is neutral to general movement. (She's fine with walking places or parking wherever, but chooses the escalator over the stairs)
✓ Jennifer dislikes intense exercise, tolerates moderate exercise, and loves light exercise.

With the following relationship scale, we are targeting everything bundled into one, considering the big picture. Based on Jennifer's profile, she'd most likely be a level 2 or 3. She isn't averse to exercise and enjoys some activities, but she dislikes intense exercise and is merely neutral in general movement preferences.

The Exercise Relationship Scale

Level 1: Strong aversion
Level 2: Some discomfort
Level 3: Neutral
Level 4: Positive feelings
Level 5: Love/addiction

Many people view exercise as Level 1:

• Intimidating

- Difficult
- Unenjoyable
- Only seen as worthwhile in large doses
- A chore (something you "should do")
- Something you dislike or even hate

Here's what exercise *can be* to you (Level 5):

- Simple and approachable
- Mentally easy to do
- Fun
- Effective and worthwhile (even in micro doses!)
- An escape in the same way that TV and video games are
- Something you crave

These two perspectives are polar opposites, and yet they refer to the exact same actions. I hope you don't grow weary of me saying it, but it bears repeating. It's all about the relationship, relationship, relationship!

For most people who struggle to exercise, the issue isn't physical ability--it's a strained or broken relationship with movement.

Thus, if you are physically able to exercise and just don't do it, you have a poor relationship with it. I don't care about laziness or how busy you are. If you love something, you make time to do it and those things won't stop you. As I said previously, I am lazy yet I now love to exercise.

If you can upgrade your relationship by even one level (i.e., level 1 to level 2), that is *significant* progress. If you can upgrade two levels, which is our goal in these 60 days, you are going to **thrive**! If you can go from level 1/2 to level 5 (which I have personally done over the years), you've won.

Warning: If you are truly at level 1, it will take time to get to level 5 (loving exercise). But just think about going from hating it to merely being neutral towards it. That's a huge leap. You will enjoy and benefit from every level "upgrade" immensely, so don't think about reaching level 5 as the only success.

Before we begin, please take a free assessment quiz about your relationship with exercise on minihabits.com/exercise-quiz.

You can take the assessment again after you finish the book, giving you a clear before/after "picture." Summer abs may come and go, but the relationship reflected in these scores determines your behavioral future.

Before We Begin

Mini Habits Crash Course

The introduction explained *what* this book is and *why* it exists. Now, we shift to *how* this is going to work. Let's start with a brief history (and time-travel) lesson.

A Brief History of Mini Habits

In December 2012, I experimented with an absurd idea to do one push-up a day. It changed my life. I systematized everything I learned, and the next year, I published *Mini Habits*. Despite my having no marketing budget and no connections, the book took off through word of mouth and is now read in 20+ languages!

The book *Atomic Habits* by James Clear has become very popular, but *Mini Habits* started this small-habit party. *Mini Habits* was published five years before *Atomic Habits*. I only mention this because a handful of reviewers have insisted that *Mini Habits* (2013) and *Mini Habits for Weight Loss* (2016) copied *Atomic Habits* (2018). That would require a working time machine. Sadly, I do not have one (yet), and if I did, I would not use it for this purpose. If I had a time machine, I would use it to help the Detroit Lions win a Super Bowl.[1]

The Core Mini Habits Idea

The *Mini Habits* premise: Instead of aiming for a big goal that you may sometimes fail to reach, aim for a smaller target that you will always be able to hit, and do it every day.

Most goals are a ceiling. A mini habit is a floor. Right now, wherever you're sitting or standing, if you could only have one, would you rather have a floor or a ceiling? A floor, I hope, because otherwise you'd be freeeeee fallllling. The same choice should be made for goals. Ambitious, high-ceiling goals are attractive, but mini habits *support* you every day. Paradoxically, the smaller my goals have gotten, the more high-ceiling goals I've been able to achieve.

What if you made success *inevitable every day*? You can do that! All you have to do is shrink your daily goal down to something "stupid small," something so small and easy that it makes you laugh and even feels a little bit insulting. For me, that was one push-up per day, and it changed my life.

Because of that daily push-up, my relationship with exercise changed. I want to guide you through the process of exactly how this works, day by day. Here's a snapshot of my relationship with exercise, in 2012 and today.

2012: Exercise was a special event. When I went to the gym, worked out at home, or went for a run, I'd feel like I did something great. Exercise was a big, weighty, high-pressure choice. It felt great to win at it and awful when I failed to do it.

2025: Exercise is uneventful. I do it every day unless I must rest. I feel good about doing it, and I enjoy it, but it's not special, it's as normal as showering. It's a lightweight and easy choice. Usually, it's my favorite part of the day!

At a glance, it almost seems as if the latter is worse, doesn't it? Exercise isn't special to me anymore. But this represents the greatest possible success you can have with any behavior, because that means it's *a normal and expected part of your life, not anything you have to fight yourself to do. It's a habit.*

A mini habit chips away at the resistance you feel toward a behavior until none remains. It really works!

This isn't just my experience, but the experience of hundreds of thousands of people. While no strategy has a 100% success rate, this one is very high. But what if it doesn't work? What goes wrong?

The greatest challenge with a mini habit is not like the challenge of most goals. Typically, the greatest challenge is the goal itself (100 push-ups, for example, require great physical effort and mental toughness to persist through them). With a mini habit, however, the greatest challenge is trusting the behavior change process and navigating your thoughts and prior goal-setting habits.

You may have thoughts like, "Why am I aiming so low? This is a waste of time." Curiously, these thoughts can persist even after seeing great success with the strategy. Before you know it, you're aiming higher and higher, risking systemic failure over a few extra reps on paper.

Extra reps are nice, and I won't pretend that they're without value. But intention and results are not always equal, and the value extra reps have is *nothing* compared to the value of consistency. Consistency is what changes the relationship. Extra reps are purely a bonus. I always encourage bonus reps, but only *as a bonus*. The idea is not to limit you, it's to ensure that you win every day. For true success, your priority must be to show up and at least do the minimum.

What to Expect

I'm going to meet you here every day for the next 60 days. Come back each day to read a short section. You can expect four types of benefits in these one-a-day pages, but not necessarily all in each day.

1. Encouragement: I'm not a "rah-rah" author, but I know how much it can help to have someone who cares about your progress. I genuinely care. I want you to succeed because I've gone through this too, and it changed my life for the better. If

that's not encouraging enough, I've added a special "reader spotlight" to some days. Mini habits have been changing lives for many years, and I've gathered some of my favorite stories and quotes from readers to share with you. These are real stories from people I've never met!

2. Guidance: You can succeed, but not if you quit on Day 4. I'm going to do my best to keep you focused on the prize. I'll remind you what the prize is and how we're getting it. If you get to the end of these 60 days, I know you'll see that everything I've said about this method is true. Then you can build upon this foundation for the rest of your life with confidence.

3. Teaching: There's a lot to learn from such a simple core idea. There are multiple "wrinkles" to discuss about habit formation and what it does for us. Since we're focused on exercise, I will include interesting facts and ideas about that, too.

4. Timing: One of the biggest drivers for me to write this book was the realization that habit formation follows a somewhat predictable path. By making this a daily book, I can give you the type of support at the time I think you'll need it most. Will the timing be perfect? Of course not! The process is the same for everyone, but the timing and individual experience will vary.

The bottom line is that I'd rather tell you an important piece of information five days before you need it than have you read a whole book once and expect you to remember a line from chapter four 53 days later when it's most relevant.

Let's Test the Theory

It's healthy to be skeptical. We live in a world where some Instagram models aren't even real people, but rather artificial intelligence creations designed with traits that people like. It's bogus. There are fake AI people with far greater social media followings than the vast majority of real, flesh-and-blood human beings. That's weird, sad, funny, awkward, and at least two more adjectives I can't think of at the moment.

In fact, many of the books you can read today are written partially or fully (!) by artificial intelligence. But absolutely not this one!

Besides, AI can't do this: *Stephen loves football and made turkey chili today!* Artificial intelligence would never say something that random, personal, and irrelevant in the middle of a book. It's too smart for that. I've written this book without AI because I think there's something valuable about the human experience and the flawed but unique communication style that AI can't replicate (yet?!).

Is the Theory Good?
Since I know this book to contain a valuable and lifelong benefit, I invite you to be skeptical of this mini habits idea. When it comes to what's good and true, scrutiny is never to be feared. The truth holds up to even the closest scrutiny.

The best way to test your skepticism is with theory first and then with observation or experience. If something makes sense in theory and you also experience it as expected, it's a winner. So here's the theory.

Mini Habits Theory: By shrinking a behavior to an easy and small level that can always be accomplished daily, we can transform our *relationship* with that behavior by making it habitual. Habits change the way we feel and prefer to act. The two critical theories that underlie this idea are:

1. Habit formation happens through consistent behavioral repetition over time (this has been proven).

2. Lowering the bar to entry increases the number of entries (also a well-known and proven concept).

The low-bar mini habit enables frequent (daily) repetition. That repetition enables brain change and habit formation. That brain change makes us like exercise more.

In theory, this works and is a good idea. In my personal experience over the last decade plus, it works better than I could have imagined. Outsized returns can also be expected here because behavioral progress and habits are *exponential*, not linear. To put that into plain terms, doing a 30-minute workout is as easy a decision today as doing one push-up was in 2012.

Who wants to spend two months to build a habit of one push-up per day? You're getting far more than that because the reps are not the true prize. New ways of thinking and a new relationship will compound your progress, and you'll easily scale the behavior up.

Bottom line: We're talking about **behavior**, meaning this must be experienced to be confirmed and believed at a deep level. Even if you are fully convinced of this idea in theory, you will never "get it" until you see it and *feel it* in practice. It's like falling in love--you can *try* to explain it, but it must be experienced to be understood in the ways that matter.

Nine Things to Know before Day 1

This is a list of nine things you need to know before you begin.

1. Know your (mini) mark for success. I recommend 1 or 2 reps of something or 30+ seconds of an exercise as your mini habit mark of success. If you want, you can make it flexible (30 seconds of *any* exercise). Or you can make it either one push-up

or one sit-up each day. Whatever you decide, be absolutely **clear** about it!

2. If you have any trouble doing your mini habit, it's one of three things: You've made your habit too large (make it smaller for decreased resistance), you don't believe it's large enough to matter (do bonus reps if you're unsatisfied on any day), or you're not making time for it (more on this in #3).

3. Because this behavior is so small, I recommend most people set a **daily deadline**, which means getting it done sometime before bed. This allows you to practice integrating exercise into your day at various times. Otherwise, you can use a set cue, such as right after you wake up, after getting home from work, after you use the bathroom, before dinner, at 7:30 p.m., before your morning shower, and so on.

4. Do your mini habit immediately before, during, or after you read that day's section in this book. Pair them together. The order isn't important. Some days you might need a little reminder of why you're doing this. That's fine--read the book first. Other days, you might want to get your mini habit completed first. Great, do that! You shouldn't *need* the book to win on any given day. This book can be what you need it to be each day--a reward (praise), a kick in the pants (motivation), or a guiding light (direction).

5. Track your mini habit. This is accountability and reward in one. Use a calendar or an app. I've also figured out a way to track it using just Kindle. To track on Kindle, simply highlight the text of "Day 1." Then attach a note describing what you did or add a simple check mark or "x." Later, you can pull up your annotations and notes for this book, and you will see each day that you've highlighted with your notes (1, 2, 3, 4, etc.). Alternatively, you can highlight or check-mark pages in the

paperback book.

6. Do the minimum (or more). Don't skip days. Skipping days is for difficult programs. You can complete some mini habits in the time it took you to read this sentence. If you miss one day, that's okay, just don't let it become two days. *Be aggressive the next day* if you miss one. One day is an aberration or small bump in the road. Two days is a new streak in the wrong direction.

7. This book is not "it's boring but it works." This is **not** only for down-the-road habits and benefits. You will notice many short-term benefits, too. Nobody will stick with something if it provides zero short-term rewards. Mini habits are more rewarding in the short term than you might think. Plus, any extra motivation you put into bonus reps feels great! It's really easy to go above and beyond when your initial requirement is essentially to show up.

8. Trust that this works. I know if you show up every day for 60 days, *really good things* are going to happen. This experience is going to surprise you!

9. Have fun. The psychology of most exercise programs is very "grindy." *Suck it up and put in the work!* Nothing makes me more eager to quit early than that sentiment. Life is "grindy" enough, isn't it? I don't need to grind when there's a more efficient, effective, and fun way to win. My workouts today might look "grindy," but that's only because I love to exercise. Make it fun now so that you can enjoy the grind later.

This is like a typical love story--it starts out as pure and lighthearted fun, and later on, it's still fun, but it gets deeper, serious, and even heavy at times. As love intensifies, there's more work involved to maintain that level of relationship. As your love of fitness grows, so will the duration and intensity of your workouts and active lifestyle. Too many programs force the issue before there's a foundational relationship to support that level of dedication. It's like asking someone you just met to marry you and being surprised when they say, "Uh... no thanks!"

Mini Habits for Fitness is a lightweight and exploratory way to get to know the marvels and benefits of exercise and increased fitness. Let's drop the lofty expectations and weighty pressures of society when it comes to fitness. Instead, we will build a healthy relationship with exercise from the ground up.

Every day, do these in any order:

- Read the day's section.
- Do your mini habit (if you want, do bonus reps).

If you enjoy this book (as I hope!), you are essentially bundling **a reward** with your mini habit, which is a nice reinforcement tool in addition to the reinforcement from the book's content.

Day 1 is next. You can start right now. You don't need to prepare for it. You don't need to be excited for it. You can't *possibly* be too busy for it. You have everything you need. Get ready to rediscover exercise in a way that feels good.

Part I

The Foundation

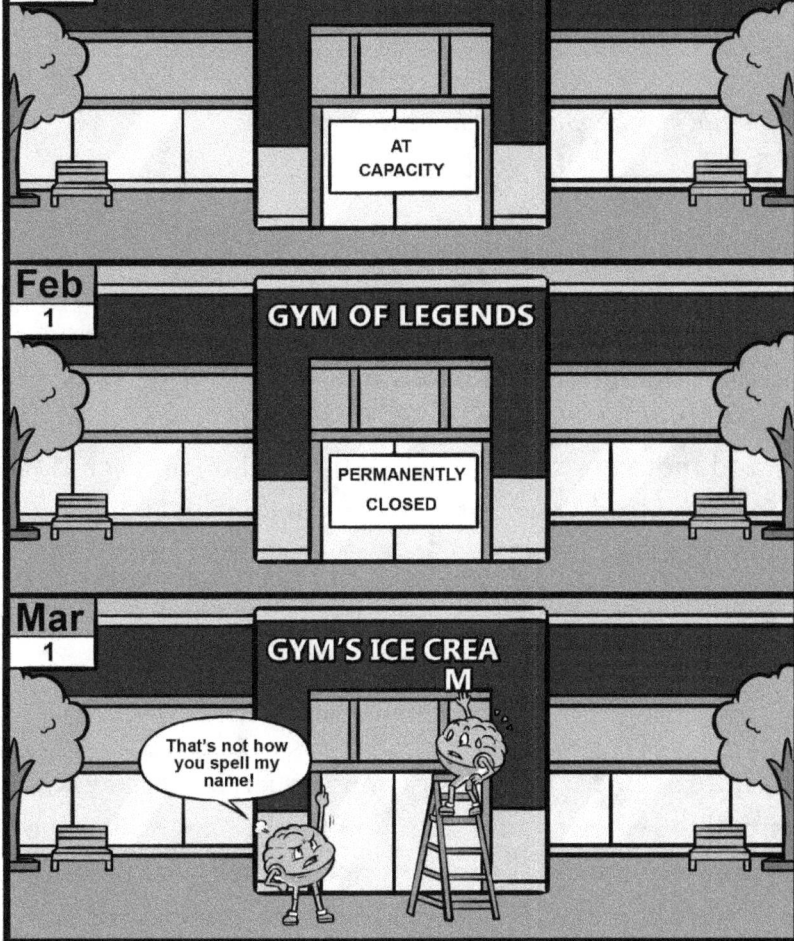

Day 1

How to Fall in Love with Exercise

"The first rule of a happy life is low expectations."

~ Charlie Munger

Do your mini habit today.

It's the first day! If you feel amped and are chomping at the bit to get going, do more. Just make sure you show up tomorrow. The mini habit keeps us on track. The bonus reps are for excess energy and motivation. On days 2-60, I will begin each day with a prompt to remind you to show up or encourage you. If you show up (even in a mini capacity), you win the day.

Reader Spotlight: "I have asthma, but wanted to start running. I started with 30 seconds a day. Five months later I was running for an hour straight 3-4 days per week... with asthma."

A small improvement in the way you perceive exercise will yield substantially greater results than you might expect. It's the kind of leverage everyone looks for but doesn't always know how to obtain. When you change the relationship, you change everything!

Example: Let's divide all of your life's moments by how much energy you have, one to five. A one would be your lowest-energy moments, like being sick, exhausted, or depressed. A five would be your highest energy moments like getting a great night of sleep or feeling inspired. For the simplicity of this idea, we'll assume you spend an equal amount of your life in each category. That means 20% of your life is lived at 1, 2, 3, 4, and 5 energy units.

Now, if you require yourself to have maximum energy to exercise (5/5), you'll only be able to exercise 20% of the time. But if you can reduce that requirement by just one unit, to four, you effectively double your odds of success. If you require three units, you triple your success rate from 20% to 60%.

Effort required: 5
Success rate: 20% (only max energy of 5 is enough)
Effort required: 4
Success rate: 40% (either 4 or 5 energy level is enough)
Effort required: 3
Success rate: 60% (3-5 energy is enough)

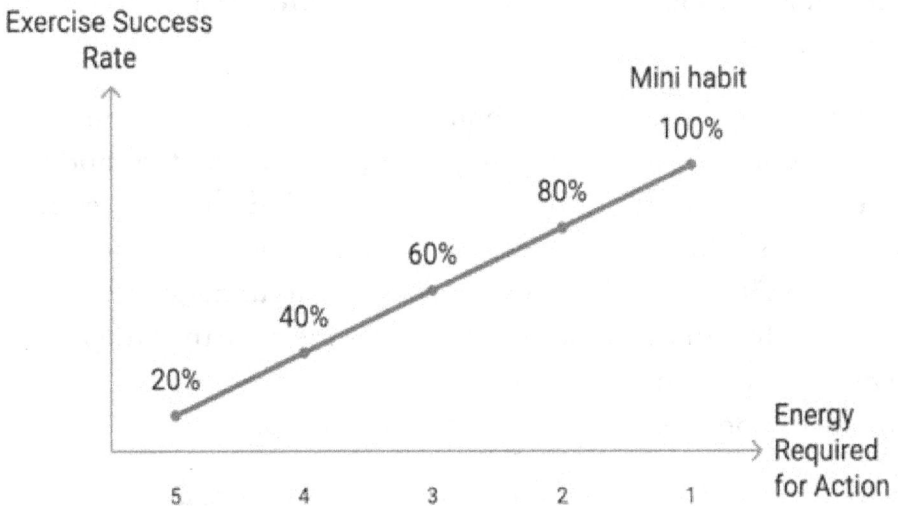

This graph shows the concept of a lower bar to entry creating more entries, but it's also an example of relationship quality, and fair warning... it might blow your mind when you see how this relates to human relationships.

One of the most important epiphanies I had writing this book is what makes a relationship healthy or not. There are numerous factors that determine how a relationship is shaped. But if you look at the end result or the snapshot status of a relationship, you'll see one thing that defines a toxic relationship.

When a relationship is toxic, anything less than perfection is perceived as negative.

Couples in toxic relationships carry resentment toward each other. Thus, any slight infraction can set them off. There's no room for error when the relationship is bad. Now picture the best human relationships in the world. What defines toxic vs healthy relationships?

When a relationship is toxic, anything less than perfection is perceived as negative.

When a relationship is healthy, imperfection is accepted with few or no conditions.

It isn't perfect behavior or chemistry that makes a relationship healthy, but the allowance of imperfection in each other and the relationship itself. Healthy relationships include flawed people doing flawed things, like the rest of us! But they are lenient with each other. They will bend over backward to understand one another. They understand that to accept their partner fully means to accept them at their worst. Their love is not conditional on their partner never messing up.

People in healthy relationships expect and require *less* from their partner.

Importantly, I'm not saying that people should unconditionally accept major character flaws or abuse in the name of a "healthy relationship." I'm merely observing how healthy relationships pan out. This is not a prescription of how to get there in a relationship; this is a fitness book using a powerful analogy we can all relate to. I can and will, however, explain how to get there with exercise, so let's switch our focus to that. The similarities are striking.

A toxic relationship with exercise demands too much. The person demands the world from exercise, and exercise demands the same from the person. We're talking about nothing but clean 30-minute-plus workouts (or perhaps one hour!). And those can only happen if it's been exactly 1.5 hours after eating, if there are no aches or pains, if traffic isn't too bad, the schedule is wide open for the rest of the day, and it's a lunar eclipse. Intense workouts are hoped for every day but only happen on those rare 5/5 days.

Now, you may not see your relationship with exercise as toxic-- that is a strong word--but the exercise relationship doesn't translate as obviously as human ones. You don't go to the gym to scream "I hate you!" at the stair machine or throw wine in a dumbbell's "face." Rather, exercise-relationship toxicity manifests subtly as avoidance, excuses, shame, and frustration. But there's good news--mending your relationship with exercise is MUCH easier than fixing a human relationship.

A small improvement in *any* relationship means exponentially more success in more situations. This improvement is seen as a gradual increase in acceptance of imperfection. A lowering of the guard, if you will.

Your mini habit is the lowest effort requirement possible. Can you see why now? This mimics a dramatically improved and healthy relationship with exercise, and we get to experience it right away on Day 1. It mirrors the loving couple who's been together for 60 years. It's a relationship without baggage or unrealistic expectations, and it's built to last.

Later, when you grow to love exercise, the physical effort component will fade into the background. The mental challenge of getting yourself to work out will become irrelevant. Instead, you'll see it as your escape, your happy place, and your therapy. It will be like the old couple, blinded to the wrinkles in their partner's face--they only see a beautiful soul. We'd all be lucky to grow old with a behavior like exercise.

Most people approach fitness by trying to maximize their energy to meet their 5/5 expectations and desired results for exercise. I understand how this seems correct at first. But this honest mistake is what prevents us from enjoying exercise and getting better results.

While a person desiring a dramatic fitness transformation may have the same fitness goals as an established fitness lover, the underlying relationship is often the opposite. When you *love* exercise, you don't struggle to do it. It's easier for me to work out for an hour today than it was to work out for five minutes 20 years ago.

Most people try to mimic sets and reps, as if following a recipe. That's not the answer. The relationship that enables consistent sets and reps is the true prize.

In a fitness relationship, you won't always be at 100% for exercise, and exercise won't always give you 100% back in return. This remains true even for elite athletes and bodybuilders but is especially prominent for beginners without a physical or mental fitness base. Fitness lovers accept imperfect energy, imperfect conditions, imperfect experiences, and imperfect results, and they still love the process. Case in point, I have a shoulder injury right now! Exercise physically hurt me, and yet I can't wait to exercise again (more carefully).

Beginners try to mimic the workload of fitness lovers but, since they don't yet love the process, they're thrown off by the slightest imperfection.

Instead of pressure for an unrealistic leap into fitness glory, let's build a healthy relationship with exercise from the ground up. In practice, that's this book. To be more specific, it means that, unlike extreme workout programs, you can still show up on bad days here, because your task is that easy.

Your choice to pursue a mini habit instead of a brutal exercise program is literally choosing a healthy fitness relationship instead of a toxic one. One push-up isn't incredible, it's small and imperfect. An extra short walk isn't maximum progress, it's just a little bit more than you're used to doing.

Imperfect progress is the bedrock of a healthy fitness relationship, and that will not change even as your abilities get more advanced.

Just like in a healthy human relationship, imperfection does not nullify the fact that what you're doing is good. *It's very good, as it allows the relationship to grow.* In time, your imperfect-but-good mindset will produce a juggernaut of profound and life-changing fitness, which includes the results you desire.

It's just as Charlie Munger said: *The key to a happy wife is low expectations.*

Wait. I messed up there. He said *life*, not *wife*. Oh, well... that too. If you require a 5/5 experience to enjoy anything, you will be frequently disappointed. This is an extra-powerful life lesson that goes beyond fitness, but I won't charge you extra.

Remember, your expectations determine success and failure more than anything else. You set the bar. Set it wisely!

Tomorrow, we'll discuss why you're ready right now.

Day 2

Why You're Ready Now

"The only way you can hurt the body is not to use it. Many of our aches and pains come from lack of physical activity."

~ Jack LaLanne

Show up today. Use your body.

Consider these two truths:

1. You're always ready.
2. You're never *perfectly* ready.

Fact #1 is empowering, but combined with fact #2 it's *even more empowering*. Remind yourself of these facts as often as possible. You don't have to wait for the right time and place to start. It's okay to have doubts. It's okay to be or feel less than your best. You can still move forward and win the day.

Many (or most?) good things in life require you to jump in before you have all the information, and certainly before you feel fully confident. These 60 days will show you how to take small steps forward within uncertainty, and the opportunities and benefits of doing it will amaze you.

Most programs: Follow step 1 exactly, then 2, 3, 4, and 5... (no autonomy)

This program: Show up. You're the boss. You decide what the

win looks like today.

The difference between following something step-by-step and this strategy is ownership. You can own your mini habit journey because your path and bonus reps will be unique to your personality, lifestyle, and challenges. You will decide when and where to push yourself and when to take the easy win.

Getting expert guidance is great. Expert guidance combined with autonomy is better. The more autonomy you have within a program or strategy, the more sustainable it is when it ends. Recipes are for cooking. Autonomy-powered strategies are for behavior change.

This is the show-up strategy. I promise you that if you show up every day, good things will happen. Consistency matters so much more in the beginning than what exercise you choose to do or if your form is perfect or if you get in X reps. You'll see why!

Tomorrow, we will discuss an interesting question. Can a habit be too small? The answer is... yes.

Day 3

Can a Habit Can Be Too Small?

"Habit is a cable; we weave a thread each day, and at last we cannot break it."

- Horace Mann

Make today count.

Yes, it turns out a habit can be too small. But it rarely is for exercise.

The only way a mini habit is too small is if it fails to start the process. For example, one reader of *Mini Habits* told me about her writing habit. She wrote one word per day and did not make much progress. I was surprised for a moment and then realized why. Writing a single word requires little thought, so it never activates the writing process. One sentence could work, since you have to think about structure and content, but I like to aim for 50 words a day when writing (about a paragraph) to ensure I get my writing gears moving.

For exercise, one push-up sounds meager, but it *does* begin the process of exercise and engages your muscles. If you feel like you need two to get you going, aim for that. Just don't pick a level that makes you hesitate. Make it so easy that it isn't a decision.

The mini habit sweet spot:

- ✓ Big enough that it starts the process.
- ✓ Small enough that you can always do it.

Put those together, and every day you will create momentum in the direction you desire. That will create powerful results in the short term and long term!

When you begin motion with a small aim, you make short-term big wins **more attainable**. In other words, starting small doesn't prevent you from finishing big. It will take time to retrain yourself to think about goals as floors (instead of ceilings). Remind yourself that your fitness mini habit is a **start** and you decide each day how far you want to go.

Tomorrow, we will discuss why you should recommit to this every day.

Day 4

Recommit Daily

"You'll never change your life until you change something you do daily. The secret to your success is found in your daily routine."

- John C. Maxwell

No human has ever lived in tomorrow. We can only ever live in today.

Reader Spotlight: "I am a mental health provider. Many of my clients have become so stuck that they feel that nothing will help them. They can't lift themselves out of depression or balance themselves out of anxiety. I have taught them what the mini habits concept (and book) can do for them, and dozens have made amazing improvements because they finally realized that life does not have to overwhelm them into despair."

Don't think of this as one big commitment; think of it as 60 mini commitments, and recommit to your mini habit each morning. You can even do your mini habits in the morning if you want to start the day with a win.

Here's why you should stick with this:

1. This really works. Trust the process. Hundreds of thousands of people have already changed their relationship with exercise, using mini habits. It's proven. (I'm one of the success stories.) This book will give you daily guidance so you

43

can do the same.

2. **This is too small and easy to skip.** Even if you have doubts, it costs you nothing to keep going today.

3. **It won't take much time or effort.** If you do the minimum, which is completely fine, you're done in seconds. *We do the minimum on some days so that we can excel on other days.*

4. **This can last a lifetime.** Most workout programs are a short-term burst of hope followed by exhaustion and a reversion to the mean. You're left demoralized and looking for answers. These 60 days are designed to improve your *relationship* with exercise. The net result of going from loathing exercise to looking forward to it is life-changing.

Tomorrow, we're busting excuses. You've got them. We all do. Most of them aren't valid, especially for an easy mini habit.

Day 5

Excuse Busters

"Watch your thoughts, they become your words; watch your words, they become your actions; watch your actions, they become your habits; watch your habits, they become your character; watch your character, it becomes your destiny."

~ Lao Tzu

Challenge your excuses. Most will fall.

You may want to reference this page later.

Wisdom is not only found in ancient tomes, because its sources are plenty; great wisdom can be found in surprising places. And on that note, instead of quoting a philosopher or scientist, I'm going to share a quote from a sitcom character.

"There are always a million reasons not to do something."

~ Jan Levinson from "The Office" (US Version)

We all know this to be true from experience. This information is especially important to our cause because we are engaging in a behavior that we're not completely comfortable with yet. Thus, you will have excuses, even for something as small and easy as a mini habit.

One of the most important secondary skills you'll build in these 60 days is responding to your excuses with simple truths. Here are a few you'll likely encounter:

Excuse: "I'm too tired."

Busted: Your chosen mini habit should be so easy you can do it while exhausted and half asleep. You're never too tired *for this*.

When I first started my push-up mini habit, I would sometimes do my one push-up in my bed. I'm not proud of that, but it worked. Mini habits are more of a psychological challenge than a physical one, which makes sense since we're targeting brain change.

In extreme physical challenges, the mind concedes first. That's why a push-up in bed--a small physical win and a big mental win--is great despite seeming subpar or even silly on the surface.

Excuse: "I don't have time."

Busted: You need less than a minute. *Everyone* has that much time, every day.

This is different from most pursuits you've ever done. Our lives are made up of one-hour appointments, 30-minute TV shows, 30-minute meetings, one-hour lunches, and so on. The concept of setting aside one minute for something is foreign to most. But that's why most people frequently choose ZERO. It's my mission to show you how much better one is than zero. It's huge. This is one of the biggest mindset shifts you'll ever make. Continue to take the mini leap of faith with me and you'll see.

Excuse: "Today is a horrible day. Something terrible happened."

Busted: A mini habit shines brightest in the darkest of days. Do the minimum and then go take care of yourself.

When tragedy strikes us, we tend to be severely weakened by it. This is the worst-case scenario, and it's exactly why a mini habit is *mini*. If we were at 100% power every day, we could set a static, high goal and crush it without fail. But life is dynamic, with some serious lows, and we want to win on those days too.

If you need to take time to grieve, or bounce back from something, that's okay. Come back to this book when you're ready. I've been there. When my dad died, I didn't care about anything for a while, including anything as easy as a mini habit. I decided to be **goalless** at that time. I had already developed an exercise habit, which helped greatly. We all handle things differently, but I know that exercise helps a lot in times of emotional stress.

A reader of the original *Mini Habits* book told me that continuing her mini habits helped her get through a tragic fatal accident of a relative. Habits can bring stability in the midst of trauma. Exercise is especially effective at moderating negative emotions, so if you can stick with your exercise mini habit in the storm, I do recommend it. Do whatever you need to take care of yourself.

Excuse: "I don't feel like doing it."

Busted: Do it anyway. Feelings will fluctuate, but this is too easy. Don't make it a decision when you can get it done so quickly. David Allen's two-minute rule in *Getting Things Done* is perfect: if it takes two minutes or less, it isn't worth thinking about whether or not to do it. Just get it done. Plus, once you start, your feelings may change and you might end up doing bonus reps. Trust me when I say these are the most satisfying and empowering wins.

Excuse: "I don't want to do something this small and meaningless. I want to do more and be more."

Busted: That's perfect. Do as much as you want today and every day of this. It's critically important to remember that your mini habit is *never* a ceiling (unlike most goals that you hit and quit). A mini habit is your *floor*, your starting point. You're always welcome to do as much exercise as you want and/or can physically do. Just make sure you also show up the next day.

By pursuing fitness the mini habits way, you will learn to prioritize daily success over raw numbers and results.

Sun Tzu famously said, "Victorious warriors win first and then go to war, while defeated warriors go to war first and then seek to win." Common fitness goals have you going to war, seeking to win, and that often ends in defeat because it's backwards. Your mini habit makes you a victorious warrior now--collect your win immediately and *then* see what more you can do.

Tomorrow, we'll talk about the ripples of action. The initial impact of a behavior is only the beginning.

Day 6

Ripples of Action

"It takes but one person, one moment, one conviction, to start a ripple of change."

~ Donna Brazile

The choices you make today ripple for the rest of your life.

Reader Spotlight: "Try it once and you will believe!"

Every successful action is like a pebble dropping into a pond. The size and number of ripples that emanate from it dwarf the initial impact. When thinking about your mini habits, don't merely focus on doing "only one push-up." Consider the ripple effect of...

- ✓ choosing to show up.
- ✓ giving yourself an opportunity for bonus reps.
- ✓ building a life-changing habit.
- ✓ improving your mood.
- ✓ impacting other areas of your life.

No action happens in a vacuum. Every action will affect your next action(s). It will affect the way you feel about your day and your life. This is why small actions carry so much weight in practice. Despite their size, they have the same ripple effect that big actions do.

My diet improved when I began exercising consistently. Being healthy in one area made me want to do it in other areas. Exercise made me feel better, and that created a natural curiosity to experiment with a better diet. Don't be surprised if you see this in your journey, too.

When I first did this, I broke free from the weight of my (and society's) unrealistic standards. Your standard in every area of your life is personal to *you*. And there's no need to feel bad about having a "lower" standard than someone else. Lower standards mean more consistent success, which builds and enables higher standards over time.

As you ditch unrealistic expectations of change, you'll see the power of living freely. Maybe you see it already. Do you see how movement (exercise) could be a lightweight and fun thing to do instead of a restrictive cage of shame?

...

I have a request for you.

Sometime between now and Day 10, the end of the first phase, try to have at least one day with the bare minimum and at least one day with some bonus reps.

Mini habits encourage bonus reps--any reps beyond your initial (mini) requirement. And I know that some people will do bonus reps each day, while others will do the bare minimum most days. Either way is absolutely fine. You will grow at your own pace. But, if you want to have the best chance of success with this system, you need to experience and embrace *both of these ways*.

Mini habit: one rep or 30-60 seconds (your floor and safety net)

Bonus reps: additional exercise (upside)

You can do the minimum and still feel okay about it. I know it looks lame on paper. But you know what looks great on paper?

A winning streak!

Small daily goals ensure you keep engaged and stay active. That is far more important than how many reps you do!

As for bonus reps, these are important too. At some point in your journey--and this will differ for every person--you're going to want to "play around" and test your limits. Self-driven exercise like this is far more valuable to your future growth than following orders.

At first, you might only do more on days you feel good. Then you might try doing a little extra on days you feel average. Eventually you will experiment with wanting to do absolutely nothing, doing your minimum, and saying, "You know what, I'm going to do more because I know I can. I'm going to get a bonus win on this horrible day."

It's on that last type of day that this strategy will truly click as *special*. When you start winning big in scenarios in which you expected to get a zero, you're doing something right. You're training to become unstoppable.

Tomorrow, we're talking about lasers. Every exercise book talks about lasers at some point.

Day 7

Lasers Can Cut through Metal

"I fear not the man who has practiced 10,000 kicks once, but I fear the man who has practiced one kick 10,000 times."

~ Bruce Lee

Practice consistently. Consistency is the key to mastery.

Reader Spotlight: "It's been so fun! I've already got a week of days X'd off on my calendar beside my bed. In addition to my mini habits, I've found myself doing lots of bonus reps, dancing regularly throughout the day, stretching, and doing jumping jacks just randomly."

When you attempt to add or improve a behavior, it's not an easy equation. Imagine that your current behaviors are a solid metal barrier, and you have to break through it to replace them. And your effort for this new behavior is represented as light.

A bright flashlight looks impressive and even seems powerful at first, but it can't penetrate a metal wall. You can shine it on the wall as much as you want without results. Put simply, the energy in the light isn't strong enough... or is it?

What if that same bright light were focused to a pinpoint? Now that light is a laser! Some lasers are capable of slicing through metal like cake. This is a valuable lesson in behavior change.

You must focus your energy and effort to succeed in behavior change.

From what we know about how the brain works, repetition over time is the only effective path to change it for the better. This tells us that our focal point must be consistency--showing up in some capacity every day. That's a mini habit.

It will be tempting to think you're "good" on Day 18 and can ratchet up your goal to 25 push-ups a day. But that is not laser-focus on the first phase of the workout (showing up). You're now spreading your focus to showing up *and* doing a decent amount. Bigger goals might feel better when you set them, but we know that a higher bar to entry decreases the number of entries. To change a behavioral relationship, you want as close to 100% success rate as possible for as long as possible.

Every day that you show up, your focused light becomes a stronger laser that gets closer to overpowering your former behaviors. It isn't so much the brightness of the light (effort) but how it is deployed in a focused way (strategy) that makes it work. Impressive numbers (I ran 5 miles today) always lose to focused consistency (I ran a little bit every day for 60 days in a row).

I know you have come into this with other responsibilities, hardships, and goals. You might even want to pursue multiple habits right now. But I ask you one thing: commit to this. Make it a priority. I don't lightly ask anyone for a commitment; I just know *what I'm asking* of you is reasonable. Easy, even.

Consistency is everything when it comes to changing your brain and how you perceive a behavior.

Tomorrow, we're going to talk about your fuel source.

Day 8

Your Fuel Source

"Forget inspiration. Habit is more dependable. Habit will sustain you whether you're inspired or not."

- Octavia Butler

Make today an 8-day winning streak.

Is it time to give up? I'm kidding. How absurd to suggest anyone would give up this early! But ask yourself *why* that's absurd, and you'll discover something interesting.

Behaviors die when we don't show up, and we don't show up when our chosen fuel source runs out.

It seems ridiculous to give up on day eight because intuitively we understand that we have the most energy and power near the beginning of a challenge. It's a simple equation:

When your power > your challenge = success

When your power < your challenge = failure

Your Source of Power

Many people use motivation as their primary fuel source, and motivation follows a predictable pattern--it starts strong and fades with time.

Others may try for a more disciplined, willpower-based

approach. Willpower is forced action, but it can fail when you don't have the energy to fight against your preferred behavior, such as watching TV (subconsciously preferred behavior) vs. using the treadmill (consciously desired behavior).

Motivation is tied to emotion--how we feel about doing something--and gets weaker as a behavior becomes less novel.

Willpower is tied to mental strength and energy--how forceful our will is--and gets weaker when we're tired or stressed.

The solution seems straightforward at first--we need to be powerful to succeed and overcome challenges. But don't forget there are *two* variables at play (our power and our challenge). We can change our *relative power* by changing our challenge to an easier mini habit.

Most try to increase their power to overcome challenges, relying on unreliable things like motivation (and dodging life's curveballs). It's smarter to decrease your challenge. In comparison to your mini habit, you're very powerful even on your worst days.

Did you know that a small goal can actually give you more energy than it requires? Larger goals require you to "muster up" willpower strength or "psyche up" your motivation to reach their high level. Small goals give you confidence because you know you can crush them.

Small goals make you feel powerful, and people who feel powerful act more powerfully than those who don't.

There's one more thing. Most people adopt a "whatever it takes" strategy for goals. They think, "I'll try to stay motivated, and if that fails, I'll force myself forward with willpower." That sounds like a great plan until you realize that the days you are low in motivation, you will be low in willpower too!

Low energy, a common goal killer, saps *both* motivation and willpower. Stress, another common goal killer, sends people running to their old habits. Simply being busy can usurp you even on days you have decent motivation and willpower.

We're choosing something that doesn't require an upbeat mood, superhero determination, or even much of our time. We just need to do one push-up (or equivalent) per day. That goal is so fuel-efficient that the government might offer a tax credit for it.

Tomorrow, we're going to talk about Day 9, why nobody respects it, and what to do about it.

Day 9

Nobody Cares about Day 9

"If I had eight hours to chop down a tree, I'd spend the first six hours sharpening my axe."

~ Abraham Lincoln

Milestones happen naturally for those who make daily progress.

It's Day 9, a day that nobody cares about because it isn't large or clean like 60 or 100. Milestones give us a target to aim for and celebrate. But let's think about what that target means. Let's think about literal targets in archery. Here are two pitfalls:

1. Imagine archery with **no target**. Pointless! You need to aim at something in order to hit it.
2. Imagine a **poorly skilled archer** with a target to hit. Not good either! An archer's skill level determines *if they are able* to hit the target.

Most people recognize that they need a target and thus avoid pitfall #1. But how many also avoid pitfall #2? To hit a target, you mustn't focus on the target; rather, you must focus on developing the skill of archery. The target serves as a useful marker of progress and skill, but, while it is necessary, it does not create success--that's your training.

I visited a bow hunting website to learn about proper archery form. I found a bulleted list with 16 points about the proper form recommended for archery accuracy. Can you guess how many out of the 16 points mentioned the target?

Zero.

Proper archery form has to do with your posture, how you hold the bow, the alignment of various markers, how you draw and release the string, and so on. I can put it like so--to hit a target, you must first become the kind of person who is able to do so. Become a person who knows how to fire an arrow with precision and consistent good form.

Of course, you can just pick up a bow and try to hit the target, but this way you will make numerous preventable mistakes. Even worse, as you continue to practice poor form, you will get better at having poor form!

When people set goals, they tend to focus intently on the target and try to do whatever it takes to get it. This is no different from the amateur archer picking up a bow and shooting relentlessly without forethought and preparation. It can work, but it's less likely to work than doing it the proper way.

This book shows the proper form of building a new behavior (exercise) into your life. The target might be weight loss, increased fitness, a better body, improved health, or all of the above. But to hit any of those targets, we must first learn the proper form of making a behavior into our habitual preference. Here's the proper form:

- **Low difficulty:** difficulty ramps up as our skill and strength do
- **High consistency:** you must practice to learn
- **Make it enjoyable:** fun habits stick faster and easier
- **Lower the stakes:** high stakes trigger avoidance (only 83%

of people get to play Russian roulette a second time)

We continue to practice this proper form until exercise does not intimidate us. It stops becoming that annoying thing that everyone says we "should do." Instead, it's simple, easy, repeatable, and increasingly enjoyable.

In time, exercise will be a highlight of your day, a challenge you enjoy (it's fun when you have the skills to meet a challenge). This is massive leverage for *any* fitness target you wish to hit. Let's do it.

Tomorrow is Day 10. I will have a special request for you.

Day 10

Please (A Request)

"Do not repeat the tactics which have gained you one victory, but let your methods be regulated by the infinite variety of circumstances."

~ Sun Tzu

Crush your mini habit today. Afterwards, notice how simple and easy it was, and remember it in case you ever think about skipping a day. It's common to forget just how easy this is.

Today is Day 10. How is your motivation? Whether high or low, your job today is to show up. Do your push-up. Walk one block. Practice yoga poses for one minute.

Even with a system as simple, easy, and effective as this one, some people will quit early. Maybe they don't believe it can work. Maybe they want to have more impressive goals on paper. Not everyone who starts a process will finish it. So here's my request to you.

Please see this through to the end. Don't do it for me; do it for yourself.

Nothing else I've tried has worked as well as this method. And I've tried everything. I once created a system with points I could buy things with--basically making exercise into currency. That was fun, but it didn't last. The results I've experienced from having mini habits have continued to serve me more than a decade after I first tried "The One Push-up Challenge" in 2012.

This will be the best effort-to-results you've ever experienced. I'm not asking you to work harder like 99.985% of fitness books will do. I'm asking you to work smarter and get on the same page as your brain. The results of this method are humble at first, but they accumulate in surprising ways.

I'm asking you to see this through right now for a reason. We're about to enter the most difficult time of this entire journey, in which the behavior begins to transition from conscious to subconscious (habit). "The handoff" begins tomorrow. Don't miss it!

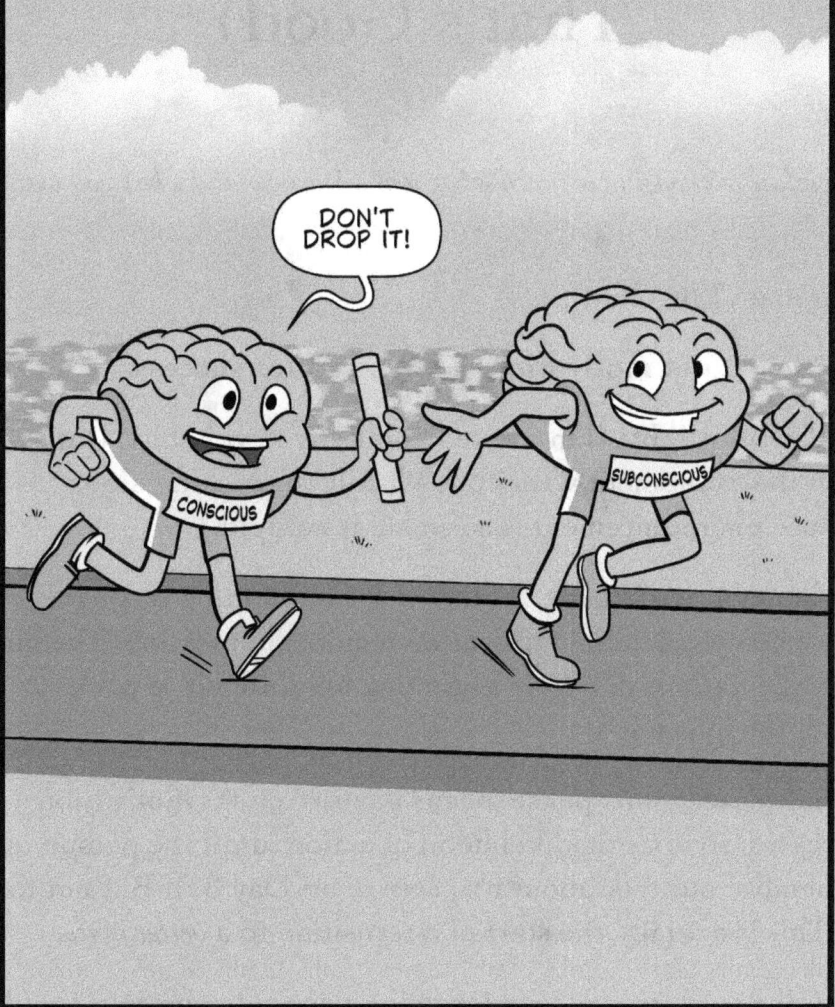

Day 11

Motivation May Wane (Why That's Good)

"Discipline is choosing between what you want now and what you want most."

- Abraham Lincoln

A decision, not motivation, is required for success.

Reader Spotlight: "I'm excited about my new habits. But even when the excitement wears off, I'll still be trucking along because the requirement is so small, it's stupid."

The honeymoon is over. By that, I mean that this is roughly the time when your initial motivation may begin to wane. The hope and expectations of a new beginning are difficult to parlay to the end of the journey.

For most goals, this phase means game over. As motivation decreases, so does the likelihood of action, until the person quits (remember our talk about fuel source on Day 8?). But not for us! This is actually the start of a transition to a *better place*.

From the start, we've been targeting your subconscious mind. We want to change the way you feel about exercise on the deepest level. Once you change that, it's easy mode. If you don't believe me, look at any "gym rat" and ask yourself if they are truly that disciplined or if maybe they just love to work out.

Nearly always, it's the latter. My brain has experienced both sides of this.

In the handoff from conscious to subconscious, a behavior becomes less exciting. It's not as easy to get psyched up about it, nor does it feel as special afterward. That's bad news for motivation but good news for habit formation. The most ingrained behaviors a person has are the least emotional. Brushing your teeth, showering, and the processes that make them up are almost mindless.

These behaviors are like vines that wrap around the core of our being. They become part of us, and so they don't surprise us, make us upset, or elate us. They just *are us*. They're unremarkable to us even if spectacular to others.

Isn't it odd that we have a drying off routine after a shower? Or that we tend to brush our teeth in the same exact pattern night after night? It's because it's more brain- and energy-efficient to do so. Thankfully, we don't need to get "psyched up" for taking a shower.

But--and this is important--the routine process and results of a behavior are still enjoyable.

- ✓ Brushed teeth? Clean mouth.
- ✓ Brushed hair? Looks nice! I'm bald, but my opinion still counts.
- ✓ Shower? Water feels great and being clean does too.

In the same way, exercise won't be a mindless and dull experience for you; it will feel incredible. Unlike the simple examples above, exercise releases all kinds of feel-good chemicals, gives you a pump (if lifting weights), and helps your whole body operate better for the rest of the day and beyond.

I know it can feel disappointing to leave the motivation phase, just as a couple feels sad to end their literal and metaphorical honeymoon. But the honeymoon pales in comparison to the importance and enduring riches of long-term success.

Tomorrow, we will tear the roof off. There's no ceiling here.

Day 12

There's No Ceiling

"Do not let what you cannot do interfere with what you can do."

~ John Wooden

Do some bonus reps today.

Reader Spotlight: "Many years ago, I stumbled upon the mini habits method--and it quietly transformed my life. Instead of chasing big, intimidating goals, I started with the tiniest actions: a short prayer, a stretch, a mindful bite. Just that. Over time, those small steps became daily rhythms. Prayer turned into a steady spiritual anchor, my eating habits grew more intentional, and movement became part of my flow. It's not about perfection, but about showing up--gently, warmly, and with love."

Extra motivation is good. Use it to exercise, not to inflate your goal size. When you are excited about making progress, it can feel strange to aim so low. Can't you do better than just one push-up?

To that thought, say, "Good. Prove it." If you can crush your mini habit, you are not only welcome to do it, you are heartily encouraged! A mini habit is not an end like most goals. Thus, you should never feel frustrated that your goal is "too small."

If you think your goal is too small, it's because you're seeing

it as a ceiling.

Your mini habit is a safety net. Your production on any individual day can be as high as you want. Just make sure you show up the next day.

It's helpful to see each day as having one mandatory goal (mini habit) and one optional goal (bonus reps). Once you meet your mini requirement, feel free to aim higher if you feel like it. **Just make sure that you don't replace the mini habit with a needlessly higher target.** The higher you jack up your floor, the easier it is to fall. High floor goals may work for a few days, but they won't likely last long enough to change your brain like a mini habit can.

To clarify, once you've completed your mini habit, feel free to then make a NEW higher goal if you wish. That is completely fine and a correct use of this strategy.

Good: I've just walked one block (mini habit complete). Now I want to walk a mile (bonus).
Good: I recognize that I only have to walk one block, but I want to walk a mile today.
Good: I walked one block. It's hot outside and I have a lot to do. I don't want to do more right now, so I'll stop there. I showed up and that's a win.
Not okay: Walking one block isn't enough. I need to walk at least a mile for it to mean something.

Setting a big exercise goal *while exercising* will always beat setting a big goal *before* exercising. You're already in motion!

Tomorrow, we will discuss why you should doubt some of your doubts.

Day 13

Doubt Your Doubt

"Doubt kills more dreams than failure ever will."

~ Suzy Kassem

You've established a successful pattern. You're building momentum.

It's normal to doubt your ability to see a long-term objective through until the end. You've just begun building a habit that you want to have for years. These days are like laying the foundation of a house.

I remember working construction one summer, and the process of preparing for a building is fascinating. We combined concrete and rebar beneath what would become the actual building. The prep work we did wasn't visible at the end, but it provided tremendous (and necessary) structural benefits. Without a solid foundation, houses and habits are susceptible to collapse when (literal or figurative) storms arrive.

The great results you achieve later will have foundational days like today to thank. Enjoy your mini habit today by thinking about its role in your long-term success. You're pouring concrete today. Later, you'll have a beautiful house of fitness. I took it too far, didn't I? "House of fitness" is not a phrase that should exist. Actually, that could be a gym name. I digress!

If you feel doubt in these days, that is normal. But I encourage you to doubt those doubts. The humble beginning stages of anything are the least impressive and most doubt-ridden. Apple started in a garage but became a modern world technology pillar.

Nobody doubts a maestro *while performing their magnum opus*. It's the earliest work that must persist through doubt to ultimately reach Magnum Opusville. Your magnum opus comes later--you can think back to this day when it comes.

Tomorrow is Day 14, the approximate day that I would often quit my goals (before mini habits). But your mini habit is too easy to quit now, isn't it? Show up tomorrow and we'll talk about it!

Day 14

Many People Quit Goals around This Time

"If you pick the right small behavior and sequence it right, then you won't have to motivate yourself to have it grow. It will just happen naturally, like a good seed planted in a good spot."

- B.J. Fogg

This is a dangerous time. Don't forget how easy your mini habit is. Stay with me!

Today marks two weeks, and studies of new year's resolutions have found that many resolutioners abandon them in about two to four weeks. There's a fitness app called Strava with hundreds of millions of activity logs from users. They found that close to 80% of users quit their January 1 resolution by January 19.[1] Welcome to the danger zone.

For a long time, I noticed this exact pattern when attempting to exercise consistently. At first, I would feel motivated, and it would always last about two weeks. Then I'd find an excuse (or chain of excuses) to quit. And it happened so reliably that I knew it couldn't have been coincidental.

Since this is such a critical juncture in your journey, I'm going to hit you with a potent piece of information that could change the way you think about many things. Today's section is slightly

71

longer, but it's worth your time.

One Thing Nobody Talks about and Everyone Needs

Self-efficacy is defined as your belief in your ability to influence an outcome. In a two-year randomized trial, baseline self-efficacy was shown to have a significant impact on exercise adoption and maintenance.[2] Nobody talks about self-efficacy. Really, when is the last time you heard anyone mention it? And yet, it is the single most important factor in creating an exercise habit. Let me explain why.

Much of what we're doing in these 60 days is reestablishing your sense of power. You must know and believe that you have the ability to influence outcomes.

It feels crazy to even type that out, because *obviously you do influence outcomes. Obviously everyone does.* There's nothing grand or even special about that claim, and yet, its power is seismic; it's responsible for every human breakthrough in history, from inventions to personal triumphs to revolutions.

Self-efficacy is something plain and unremarkable that makes us powerful if we have it and *dormant* if we don't. Many people don't have it, but, importantly, it isn't their fault. It isn't some weakness of theirs. It's a common misunderstanding. This is how it happens.

How to train yourself to believe that you **can't** influence outcomes (low self-efficacy):

1. Pursue a difficult exercise plan (or other goal).
2. Fail at any point in that journey.
3. Notice "I tried and couldn't do it."
4. Your self-efficacy is now decreased.
5. Repeat as necessary until self-efficacy is fully depleted.

As you repeat that cycle, you will start to believe that trying itself is futile. *Can I actually influence outcomes?* You keep trying to do something and failing to do it. It seems logical to wonder if your effort matters at all if said effort doesn't produce results. Attempts decrease, defeatism sets in, and self-efficacy is all but dead. This is a horrible cycle, and I speak from experience.

But I will prove to you that the problem has never been with you or your effort level with the next three questions.

1. Does everyone have choice? Yes.
2. Do said choices influence outcomes? Yes.
3. Would a person who knows and believes this take action immediately and frequently? Yes.

Yes, we can choose, and yes, that choice has power to influence outcomes. The issue then, is found within the third question. Something is wrong with the "know and believe" part of the equation.

What prevents us from making powerful choices to better ourselves?

Self-efficacy isn't merely the power to choose and influence outcomes; it's *your belief* in that fact. Number three above shows the gap between the power people possess and their lack of belief (or knowledge) in that power. There are a *lot* of people who want things that they continue to **choose not to pursue day after day**, and fitness is at the very top of that list as the most desired change/resolution for humanity.

This means something truly heartbreaking. Many people genuinely don't believe in themselves, in their power to influence the trajectory of their lives. After numerous efforts fail, you might think you need to *try harder* and do something extraordinary to get over the hump. But you don't need to have extraordinary willpower, effort, or a personal trainer to succeed here.

To put it clearly, effort is only relevant after the choice has been made to try in the first place. That is why choice is where true power lies, not effort, as many people believe.

We don't need to try harder; we need to empower ourselves to choose the right behaviors consistently.

In reading this book, you've taken an important first step to powerful self-efficacy, but this isn't the finish line. People buy exercise books all the time in hopes to figure out how to get fit. In this book, the best answer is your experience in these 60 days.

We're inundated with messages that oversimplify behavioral psychology and neuroscience into "you gotta want it" and "try harder." I want you to remember this in regards to all of your previous failed attempts to exercise consistently: You have never been the problem. The fact you're reading this now tells me *you are trying and you do want it.*

Believing that you're the problem is the problem, because it kills your self-efficacy.

In the original *Mini Habits*, I said that people are quick to blame themselves and slow to blame their strategies. When an exercise plan fails, do you think, "I should've kept going, done XYZ, etc."? That seems harmless and even constructive, but it is incredibly damaging as you are blaming yourself.

Self-blame happens as a tragic, ironic twist of self-belief gone wrong. We've seen other people succeed with extreme workout programs. So there's no excuse, right?

If person X succeeded with this, then I should be able to, too.

But what if person X succeeded **despite** their chosen strategy, and not because of it? What if person X had already built up the specific skill(s) needed to enable their success? Our pride gets in the way here, because we want to believe we're good enough to do it, even if it's the hard way. But here's something I've learned: The hard way is romanticized, and rarely the best path. The easier way is also known as the smarter way.

The hard way is portrayed as honorable and tough (romanticized) and the easy way as cowardly and weak. That's inaccurate. The idea is that the hard way hardens you, and the easy way softens you. While there is some truth to that, it is only relevant after you've built a foundation.

Think of the hard way and easy way not as separate paths for strong or weak people, but as multipliers of your effort. The hard way gives you a 0.5x return on your effort and the easier (smarter) way gives you 2x. So however hard you try, the easier way gives you a better return. Here's a real-world example.

The hard way: Save $100 a month to get $24,000 in 20 years

The easy way: Invest $100 a month in the stock market to get $68,730 in 20 years (at the historic 10% average annual return for stocks)

Total Savings

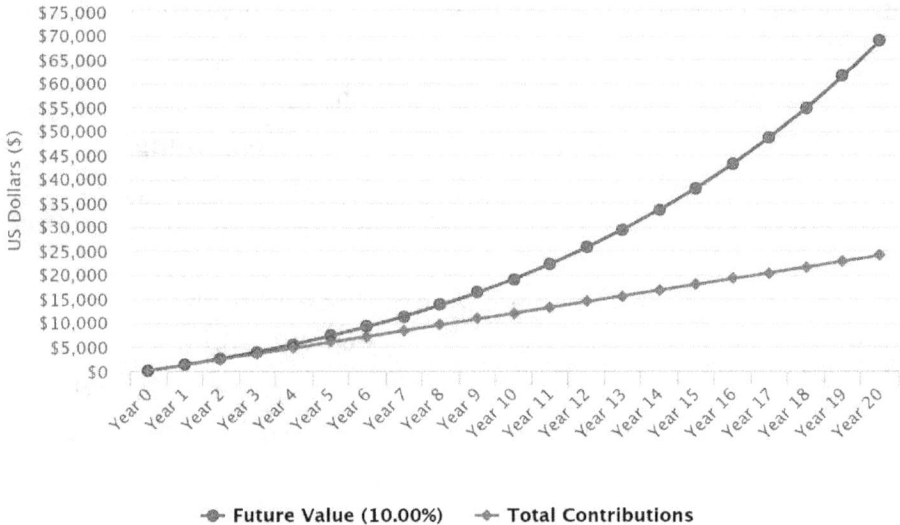

US Dollars ($)

Legend: Future Value (10.00%) — Total Contributions

investor.gov

The hard way makes you 3x poorer with the exact same earnings. Can the hard way work? Absolutely! Is it for most people? Absolutely not. It's a worse return on investment, whether we're talking about fitness effort or saving for retirement.

Common Thought: *If I try to exercise every day, and I don't do it, I have failed. I'm the problem. I know it's hard, but I need to try harder because it's important.*

Truth: *If I try to exercise every day, and I don't do it, I must change my approach. Exercise is a **simple choice** that I'm not making. There must be a way that enables me to succeed in this.*

We've already established that we can influence outcomes by choice. Thus, the only thing that can stop us is not making the choice itself. Why would a person ever choose not to exercise?

Every time I've failed to exercise, it has been because the options I gave myself were too difficult and/or unappealing. EVERY TIME.

I'm lazier than most people. I want to play games all day. I have the willpower of a salted snail. But none of that mattered when I adopted this strategy that leveraged my power of choice. I made it as easy as possible to choose to exercise and, just like that, I have now grown to love exercise.

So let me ask you:

1. Are you human?
2. Do you have choice? (Don't get philosophical on me now.)

If you said yes to those, you have everything it takes to change your relationship with fitness, get into the best shape of your life, and experience the zillions (or so) benefits that exercise gives us. These 60 days will build your self-efficacy to a level you've never known.

Look at your mini habit through the lens of this message. You aren't avoiding hard work with a mini habit, you are leveraging your power of choice and multiplying the fruits of your effort. In addition, you are learning to enjoy a new behavior and building a foundation to make hard workouts feel easy later. (When I say "feel easy," I only mean in terms of your mental attitude toward intense exercise. A strong and trained mind enjoys what would previously annoy.)

Tomorrow, we'll discuss the two stages (or phases) of a workout, and why one matters more than the other.

Day 15

Two Stages of a Workout

"Start by doing what's necessary; then do what's possible; and suddenly you are doing the impossible."

~ Francis of Assisi

Do your mini habit today. This is the first stage of any workout.

There are two stages to a workout, and it's wise to separate them.

Most fitness psychology is unilateral in thought. In other words, people think of a 30-minute workout as one event. But in the development of an active lifestyle, it's crucial to break this event into *two phases*. The first phase (our focus) ensures your success in building the habit, and the second phase drives the results that you desire from fitness.

The first phase of any workout is a simple idea: Show up. If you always show up, you will change the way you think and feel about exercise.

Consider this: If you do something every day...

- it's the definition of normal.
- it isn't intimidating.
- it feels natural.
- it's a core part of your life.

78

Think of how much *easier* it will be to exercise with that sort of relationship. That's what everyone strives for when *starting* a fitness pursuit. But this is one of the few strategies that is specifically designed to *get you there* (as opposed to assuming you're already there).

The second phase of that 30-minute workout is the raw volume: the reps, time, and effort you put in. **This is secondary and should be treated as such.** I go to the gym for one-hour weightlifting sessions, tracking all my weight lifted, sets, and reps. That's only possible because I mastered phase one with my one-push-up-per-day mini habit over 10 years ago. Even with an advanced workout regimen, showing up remains the most important part. It makes the rest of it possible.

It's true that exceptional results will only come from hours of exercise effort, but you won't do it without a reliable habitual base. Just like the foundation of a house or the under-the-surface mass of an iceberg, the unseen portion supports the seen portion.

Example: Say your mini habit today is 10 jumping jacks, and you go on to do 100 jumping jacks. Obviously, the 90 extra jumping jacks are going to have a bigger impact on your fitness than the initial 10. But the initial choice to do jumping jacks at all (the first 10) will always be the secret sauce to getting those extra 90, both today and 10 years from now.

Tomorrow, we're going to have an important discussion about Goodhart's law, how it's broken by most goal-setters, and why that kills goals.

Day 16

Respect Goodhart's Law

"Any observed statistical regularity will tend to collapse once pressure is placed upon it for control purposes."

~ Charles Goodhart

Even if you double your mini habit, it's still too easy to say no.

The quote above is the origin of Goodhart's Law, while the following is perhaps a more digestible summarization of it by Marilyn Strathern[1]: "When a measure becomes a target, it ceases to be a good measure."

British economist Charles Goodhart uttered his now-famous law in reference to the UK's monetary policy in the 1970s. Exciting stuff, I know. Since then, however, it has proven to be a universally poignant idea. Broadly, it means there is great danger in focusing too intently on specific targets, because, in doing so, we may forgo equally important things as we pursue this one variable at all costs.

Here's Goodhart's law applied to goals: Say you decide you want to lose 40 pounds in four months, whatever it takes. In this case, 40 pounds is your one measure, and you have made that measure your singular target. This is precisely what Goodhart's Law warns against. Let's break down why.

If this single measure of 40 pounds lost is your target, you will naturally optimize for it. It's this optimization for one measure that creates problems. When you optimize for 40 pounds of weight loss in four months, you'll **neglect** factors (other "measures") such as your physical health, brain change, muscle gain, sustainability of your results, happiness, metabolic health, and so on.

If one measure is your only target, you will sacrifice other valuable measures to achieve it. You will manipulate whatever you can to reach the goal, even if it creates a worse overall and even counterproductive result.

Bodybuilders have one goal--to have the best-looking body. To do that, they go through horrific and even dangerous dehydration before their show to get that shredded look. It's a good example of how surface appearance can be deceiving. Many bodybuilders have died from preparing for a show (let alone steroids).

I understand why some people might value the number on the scale above all else, but consider these...

1. Body composition: As you work out more, you may gain muscle, which weighs more than fat. The scale might not change even as you're losing fat. You can get stronger and healthier and look better without losing weight.

2. Health: Good health and healthy weight are usually synergistic. One leads to another. But many people will sacrifice their health to try to meet weight loss goals (weird diets/ starvation), which is counterproductive. The primary reason a moderate weight is desirable and more attractive to others is because it represents good health. But if you get there through unhealthy means (we don't want *Meth Habits for Weight Loss*), there's nothing to celebrate. We can and should pursue good health and proper weight *together*.

3. Mental health: Your methods will affect your mental health. If they are extreme, destructive, or induce shame, you will worsen your mental health. Your mental health is just as important as your physical health.

You could argue that how you look in the mirror is a better target than your weight. What about that as a singular target? While it is better, it still misses the mark for two reasons.

1. External appearance is not a fully reliable indicator of health. A 20-year-old bodybuilder recently died after a show due to dehydration.[2] As mentioned earlier, when bodybuilders prepare for a competition, they purposely dehydrate their bodies to look leaner. This makes their muscles pop in incredible definition, but it comes at the cost of their health until they can hopefully safely rehydrate. If the mirror becomes your only guiding light, you may be tempted to sacrifice mental and physical health and take shortcuts to get there. This is not a desirable path. Health is wealth!

2. Invisible progress: Mirror progress is the *last to show*; many positive changes won't be visible at all. For example, fat is stored all over the body, and some of it is not even externally visible. You might be looking at your stomach and feel discouraged when you're losing internal fat around your organs and/or gaining muscle elsewhere. Fat stored around the organs is the most dangerous to human health, so losing internal fat is worth celebrating, even if you can't see it right away.

The scale and mirror are the most common measures made into fitness targets. And certainly, these are very important data points. But it's better to **have a wider variety of measures** to gauge your success. Use the scale, the mirror, your energy level, your mood, your strength, your endurance, and your behavioral sustainability together as indicators of progress and success.

When you're truly doing well, these will all improve together.

Having a wider range of targets for your fitness is not only smarter and healthier; it will keep you far more encouraged throughout the journey. More targets means more opportunities for success. On the road to getting fitter, we have *many* targets to hit and feel good about!

- Are you enjoying it?
- Is your physical health improving?
- Is your mental health improving?
- Are you sleeping better?
- Do you have more energy?
- Are you consistent/building a habit?
- Does your new behavior seem sustainable?
- Do you look better in the mirror?
- Are you losing weight?
- Are you gaining muscle?
- Is your confidence higher?
- Are daily tasks like climbing stairs easier?

This is not a comprehensive list. There are countless measures of fitness success. Considering **all** of these measures in aggregate gives us the clearest picture of all we're accomplishing. Focusing on only one of these will blind you to a greater overall achievement or, worse, blind you to the harm you're doing.

A mini habit will not change the scale as much as an extreme fitness program will in the first month or two, but your small behavior will smash those programs when it comes to enjoyment, sustainability of results, confidence-building, habit-building, and long-term success. We're trading the one target (mirror or scale) for a dozen or so targets.

Remember: When a measure becomes a target, we optimize

for it (and only it) at the cost of everything else.

Make sure you don't think about your mini habit as people think about most goals. Your mini habit is not just a target to hit; it's your safety net, confidence builder, spark, and the key to a better relationship with fitness. It's a philosophical shift in how to approach exercise.

Bonus reps are an important part of this mental shift. Hit your target and use that momentum to help you climb to the bigger fitness achievements that you desire. Be curious about your capabilities. Explore them in this free and unrestricted space. You're not doing push-ups or running laps to meet an overbearing and arbitrary goal, you're pushing yourself because you want to see how far you can go and because you've seen improvement doing this every day. Which one sounds more empowering to you?

Nice job for completing today. I'll see you tomorrow. We'll talk about shame and why removing it from your life is a game changer.

Day 17

No Shame Game

"Shame corrodes the very part of us that believes we are capable of change."

~ Brene Brown

Compare your ability to the challenge of a mini habit, and you will feel strong. Those who feel strong tend to act like it.

Let's talk about shame.

Shame is feeling bad about yourself or your actions. It's poison to the mind; it has no place in your life. Shame tells you that you're not good enough, that something is wrong with you. In theory, this is supposed to provoke action. But there's one big problem with that.

Shame so often fails to incite action because it weakens us. We must act from strength in order to sustain a behavior.

Shame is a self-directed attack on the mind; it decreases your self-esteem, self-efficacy, energy, and motivation. All of those are powerful instigators of exercise! We need them.

Important: Most people think of fat shaming when it comes to shame. That's shame in regards to how you see your body or how you feel others see you. But a more hidden source of shame is the feeling that you can't physically do "enough."

When you're out of shape, your low fitness level limits what you're able to do initially. If you feel bad about this (shame), that sense of weakness seeps into your psyche and makes you quit. But if you accept that *it's okay to be where you are and that you can improve from there*, you will, I promise you, surprise yourself with how far you can go and how rapidly you can improve.

I have good news, and I hope you are already feeling this from our discussions. In these 60 days, you can destroy your sense of shame. People only hold on to shame because they don't know of another way. They might think that shame is the best way to get themselves to do something. All it does is drive them into the ground.

You've exercised 17 days in a row. That's what *elite athletes* do. Sure, they have more advanced workouts than what we're doing, but you share the same **framework of consistency** that enabled them to reach elite status in the first place. Be proud of that!

You exercise every day.

You can feel good and feel inspired by what you've already accomplished. And if you feel that right now, compare that feeling to that of shame. Which one makes you **feel more powerful**? Which one gives you **the spark of hope** that you are strong enough and have what it takes? Which one makes you want to continue making progress?

Any person can find a reason to feel shame. Any person can also find a reason to be proud of their efforts. You make this choice every day. Your mini habit is the psychological key to understanding that consistency is more valuable than raw effort.

Let today be the day that you say goodbye to shame forever. You have been moving in the right direction for more than two weeks. Leave those old ways of thinking in the dust. Forgive yourself for prior mistakes. *Allow yourself and your body to be where you are*. You're getting better every day now; you're building something to last, and you can feel good about that.

I know it's even easier to feel proud of your progress when you have visible and physical results, too. That's why tomorrow is a short but mind-blowing idea about exercise. It will help you to see how fitness progress can be exponential.

Day 18

Exponential Considerations

"Compound interest is the eighth wonder of the world. He who understands it, earns it; he who doesn't, pays it."

~ Albert Einstein

Another win is within your grasp today. Will you take it?

Reader Spotlight: "I am a 49-year-old man living in Japan. When I read *Mini Habits*, my weight was over 118 kg. First, I reviewed my diet, improved my physical condition, and eventually lost weight to 65 kg. Now I weigh around 75 kg to 78 kg, but I am gradually realizing the power of changing my habits."

Once you grow a habit of any size, it becomes a powerful floor (a new, higher standard). Not only will it prevent you from slipping into dreaded "zero" days, but a higher floor can be leveraged for exponential growth through multiple means.

Most people start with a zero floor. They go as high as they can for as long as they can, but when they aren't perfect, they get zero. They quit. And the moment you quit, you miss out on the exponential returns of exercise.

Consider this: Exercising increases your capacity for exercise. This is an exponential formula--better fitness fuels better fitness (which fuels better fitness). In addition, proficiency creates a greater incentive and reward for engaging in the behavior. Put another way, we enjoy what we're good at, so as your skill, strength, and endurance improve, so will your enjoyment of exercise.

It's well known in finance that when you're dealing with exponential formulas, you don't need a very large amount to start. You just need enough time and consistent activity for the formula to work its magic. For example, a penny doubled every day for 30 days becomes over $10 million.

The existence of exponential growth means that vanity goals can go jump in a river. We're staying small to leverage exponential growth. This works better than big goals because big goals don't keep you in the game long enough to harness exponential power.

Tomorrow, we'll talk about the many reasons that extreme programs are almost always short-lived.

Day 19

Why Extreme Never Lasts

"There is no elevator to success, you have to take the stairs."

- Zig Ziglar

Today marks 19 steps forward. That's multiple times more than any human can leap in a single bound.

Extreme exercise programs are roughly 99.99584% of the exercise market. If you're not bleeding by the end of the workout, you need to step it up! I've tried them myself, and while they're probably better than chain-smoking, they have five serious issues.

The Five Follies of Extremes

1. They threaten the brain

This is the absolute worst part of extreme workout programs. Any extreme behavior change is a significant threat to the subconscious brain's current preferences. Essentially, this means you're picking a fight with your current way of life, which is theoretically correct but neurologically unlikely to work unless the behavior has an unusually strong immediate reward (drugs).

The conscious mind is powerful in the short-term, but it doesn't have the lasting energy efficiency of the subconscious habit system. That's why so many people can override their current habits for a couple weeks or so before tiring out and going back to them.

Extreme exercise programs are a major threat to the brain of a sedentary person. But the saying goes: "You can catch more flies with honey than vinegar."

Instead of picking a fight, we're respecting and working with current subconscious preferences. We respect that we have developed some lazy habits over the years that have their own appeal and benefits. In doing so, we don't threaten that old way of living, we gradually sculpt a new way of living. The day-to-day change is almost imperceptible, and that's by design. That's what makes it nonthreatening. When difficult days arrive, we can still enforce our gentle lifestyle improvements without a problem.

2. They exhaust your energy supply

Extreme exercise programs for out-of-shape people make sense in theory. But in practice, people aren't physically and (certainly not) mentally prepared for them. Their bodies struggle to handle that amount of work, and exhaustion fatigues them mentally as well.

Even if you push through successfully, overtraining can lead to dehydration, heat exhaustion, heat stroke, vomiting, injury, emotional and mental problems, illness, extreme fatigue, insomnia, and more. Such problems are most likely to happen to an untrained person doing the most extreme exercise.

If you overcome the pain *and* serious complications of overtraining, it can simply wear you out over a number of sessions. This is generally what happens after exercise, but the degree to which you're worn out is crucial. If you really burn yourself out, it might take several days or even weeks to recover your strength. Even elite athletes know to rest when needed!

It's important to be consistent and slowly build your endurance and capacity for exercise.

3. They are unappealing

Extreme exercise for a novice exerciser can feel like torture. It's not fun to push yourself that far beyond your comfort zone. This is not to be confused with pushing yourself (a good thing!). It's all about the degree to which you're pushing your body.

I don't know if this is controversial, but I hate vomiting. Vomiting is one of the worst feelings and experiences I've experienced. Thus, any action that makes me vomit is one that I avoid (I iz smart). Due to a few food poisoning incidents, I'm very careful with food dates and storage now. You know where I'm going with this. Exercising to the point of vomiting (a common occurrence with sudden extreme exercise) would not make me want to come back to it!

As you build up your fitness level and exercise habit to high levels, you will find extreme fitness challenges to be more appealing and even fun. We are training ourselves to tolerate, then be neutral, then enjoy, and finally love fitness. Generally speaking, extreme physical challenges aren't very enjoyable until very late in this process.

4. They are unsustainable

Maybe you buck the trend and are fine with exercising until vomiting. You push through the pain and haven't overtrained. Your next issue is in sustainability. Extreme exercise is not something people (not named Goggins) can or should do daily-- this makes it more challenging to make into a habit. It's better to develop the habit first, and then leverage your habit into extreme exercise opportunities, which you can safely rest from, knowing you'll be back as soon as you're ready.

5. They don't fit everyday life

Life is unpredictable. Some days will be much busier than others. Extreme exercise plans are simply more likely to fail than what we're doing because they take more time. So even if you avoid all of the other pitfalls somehow, "life happens" can get you.

With such a small habit, you can fit it into your worst days and go for bonus reps on days you feel good and have more time. As Sun Tzu says, "Do not repeat the tactics which have gained you one victory, but let your methods be regulated by the infinite variety of circumstances." Life presents us with an infinite variety of days. It's best to be prepared for the worst but also be able to capitalize on a good day.

Tomorrow, we'll discuss simple and complex. There is a time and place for each, and it's crucial to get it correct.

Day 20

Simple vs Complex

"As simple as possible, as complex as necessary."

~ Jon Daiello

Do your mini habit today unless you are in outer space.

A daily mini habit is as simple and easy as exercise can get. But advanced bodybuilders will split workout days between muscle groups and plan out intense, precise programs full of dozens of different exercises to maximize their results. Which one is better?

Thinking in this way is the problem. Neither of these is better; it's a question of ability and need. Mini habits are better for a beginner or someone who doesn't enjoy exercising! Don't even think about advanced exercise programs if you're not automatically in the gym multiple days a week.

If you haven't established exercise as a core part of your daily life, you need to train for that objective first, and that training is simple (this book).

Fitness spans from ultra simple to extremely complex. For example, you can lift weights for hypertrophy, strength-building, and/or stamina. You'll get some of each, but different weights, sets, reps, and techniques can prioritize one over the other. There are techniques such as lengthened partials, in which you focus your exercise on the lengthened state of the muscles (eccentric) instead of the full range of motion (concentric and eccentric). There's training with restricted blood flow. There's training with masks that simulate being at high altitude.

The variety of possible techniques, exercises, and more is overwhelming. And yet, the simplest of exercises can get you very far. How about... walk more. What's simpler than that? And yet, people have lost hundreds of pounds doing *only that*.

This is how the process should look:

1. Make exercise habitual/normal/expected (mini habit).
2. Increase volume (robust habit).
3. Specialize (maximize results).

Most programs you'll find assume you are already at step three, perhaps because they are most often made by people who are at that stage and can't relate to an untrained brain. And while you can find some success with any exercise program, a lack of foundation (step 1 and 2) will make those results short-lived. Every attempted fitness cycle is discouraging because it means you haven't yet found a lasting solution. We're changing that right now!

Tomorrow is the beginning of the biggest test. You've already started the handoff, and good job making it this far, but we are still in the most challenging days of your brain transition. I call the next 10 days "the big test."

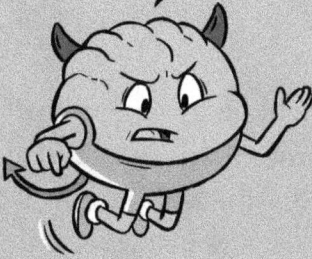

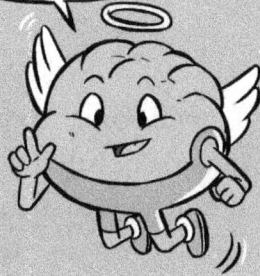

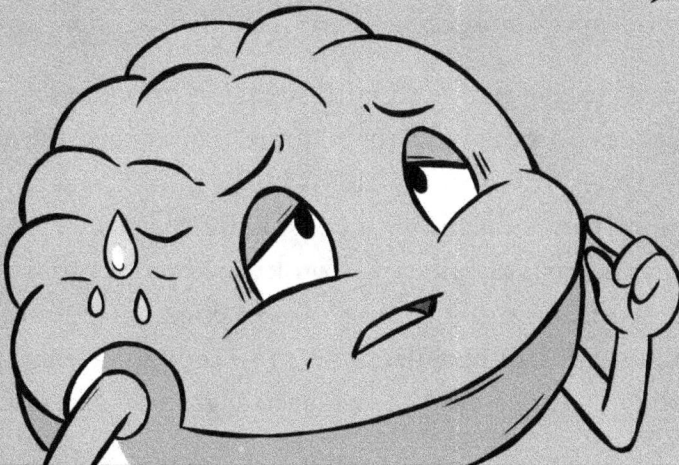

Day 21

Keep it Fresh

"You don't know what your abilities are until you make a full commitment to developing them."

~ Carol S. Dweck

Day 21 Checkpoint: Every 20 days will be a checkpoint. This is when you can slightly increase your mini habit target. But I want you to know that the reason to do this is 95% psychological. You do not *need* to increase your target unless you feel like you psychologically need to do it.

It feels good to get stronger, and this is an opportunity to put your progress on paper. There's some risk/reward here. The equation comes down to the slight boost in perceived progression from a larger goal versus the slight increase in difficulty (and risk of failure). You know by now that your goal on paper is a floor, not a ceiling. We're considering a target increase now mostly because it's fun to recognize that a bigger target today is as easy as the smaller target you started with.

You can keep your mini habit the same size, but if you feel like a greater feeling of progression might energize you, increase your mini habit today. Keep your habit very small, such as increasing from one push-up to two push-ups, or from 30 seconds to 45 seconds or one minute. (Note: If you increase your mini habit and find yourself feeling resistant, simply move your mini habit back to where it was.)

At this point, I can say with confidence that your subconscious is well aware that you've exercised for 20 days in a row. Congratulations on that, by the way. Like your brain, we don't count reps, we count days.

Stale Commitments

You're 20 days away from the day you decided to do this. I call this a "stale" commitment, because as time goes on, you get further and further away from the moment, circumstances, and person who decided to make a change. Commitments, like bread, are best right after they're made.

A stale commitment can make you feel less committed, just because it's that far from the time you made it. Since we are doing mini habits, remember that we're all about the *daily commitment*. Don't think of this as one big commitment, but 60 mini commitments that we make fresh every morning... like bread. Sorry, I'm hungry.

I call these next ten days "the big test" because this isn't new or novel anymore, and in your brain, this is a weak habit at most. **For people who use their feelings as a guide, this can mislead them into thinking that the plan isn't working.** It's working, trust me! I've been through this. And I can prove to you that excitement and feelings wane around this time.

When I first did the one push-up challenge (the challenge that evolved into the first *Mini Habits* concept and book), I noticed something peculiar in my notation.

In the early days, I would mark all of my bonus reps with encouraging phrases, and lots of exclamation points!!!! But about 20 days into it, I just started writing a check mark. Even when I'd do extra reps, I'd just put a check on my tracker. I was a bit disappointed and confused, but I shouldn't have been.

A loss of enthusiasm is what we *want* to happen! This is what habits look like. How unfortunate that so many people mistake this great sign of success for "something's wrong." I can't imagine how many goals have died because of it.

But now you know. Embrace this awkward time and enjoy the nascent normalization of your new lifestyle. Everyone has experienced the initial excitement and subsequent fading of their goal. Fewer have experienced and learned to push through these counterintuitive changes that come with new habit formation.

Tomorrow, I'm going to teach you a method that will NEVER fail. You'll want to keep it and use it for the rest of your life.

Day 22

The Neverfail Technique

"There will be very few occasions when you are absolutely certain about anything. You will consistently be called upon to make decisions with limited information. That being the case, your goal should not be to eliminate uncertainty. Instead, you must develop the art of being clear in the face of uncertainty."

~ Andy Stanley

As you do your mini habit today, notice how the decision to act is quite often harder than the act itself. That's why we make it easy to decide.

Reader Spotlight: "The mini habit takes some time to get set into one's psyche, but it works every time it is applied."

If thinking about your mini habit (or any other goal) makes you feel overwhelmed, do the following and I promise it will work *every single time*. Every time! But you have to actually do it and be intentional about this specific process.

Any moment you feel overwhelmed and paralyzed, it means you are trying to pack in too many steps and/or expectations into something that needs to be very small and easy.

Step One: identify the next project or goal you wish to make progress on. You must choose a single one.

Step Two: focus your mind on the very next physical action you need to perform to move forward. Drop any expectations and weight you may feel. Just focus on the simple action that would bring you a little bit closer to your goal. This might mean standing up, opening a book, putting on gym shorts, walking to the sink, taking one step toward your garage, and so on.

Once you take this first step, watch how your prior sense of overwhelm is superseded by forward momentum towards your goal.

There's nothing more motivating than being in positive forward motion. People tend to seek motivation to take action, when they should instead take a small action first in order to generate motivation to continue.

If you face additional resistance, you can continue taking small steps in the same direction and you will succeed. I realize how ridiculous this may sound, but you have to try it. Most people continue to wallow in impossible and bloated expectations without ever moving forward *a little bit* to see what happens next. The more you do this, the more your eyes will be opened to how powerful momentum is.

Recap: clarify your objective and take the next small action to move forward. Continue as necessary until you're in the zone.

Tomorrow, I'm going to share some thought training. This is one of my favorite methods for personal growth. We'll target and replace certain thought patterns with better ones, as if we're using the "search and replace" tool in a word processor.

Day 23

Thought Training

"Change your thoughts and you change your world."

~ Norman Vincent Peale

Today is one brick. No single brick is impressive, but together they can create a magnificent building. You need each individual brick!

The way you think about fitness has a lot to do with the internal language you use. Be careful not to use language that frames exercise in a negative light, trivializes small amounts of exercise, or makes it difficult to get started. Here are some examples of challenging thoughts you may have, with suggested reactions.

Situation: I don't think one rep is enough to matter.

Think: "All motion is valuable. Consistency is everything."

Remind yourself of this as often as possible. One rep moves you in the direction you want to go. Life isn't about the numbers; it's your direction of motion that takes you where you want to go! Added to this, consistency changes you and nothing else does. Raw numbers and reps will always matter less than *consistent successful days over time*.

Situation: I'm debating how many reps to do today.

Think: "I'll get started and figure it out as I go."

Many people have been trained to pursue goals in the following manner.

1. Set target.
2. Meet target.

This is fine and works for most things, such as doing the dishes. But when you have a more nebulous goal such as "get in shape," "stay fit," or "lose weight," you don't need specific targets. In fact, specific targets are usually worse than the decision to start. When you choose to begin with the smallest step, you minimize the difficulty of starting (the hardest part) and maximize your momentum. It's truly a win-win!

Don't get bogged down in the details. Start, get the victory, and let your momentum help you out. A person in motion will be more motivated than a person who hasn't started yet. Get moving and magic happens.

Situation: I've done my one rep. Now what?

Think: "That's a win. Do I want to do more?"

This is the thought you can use after meeting your easy requirement.

"That's a win" reaffirms your commitment and respect for consistency. You don't need to put up gaudy numbers or have your best workout ever. You don't need to feel strong, fit, or powerful every time. But you do need to show up every day in some capacity, and this thought rewards you for doing so!

"Do I want to do more?" This thought leaves the door open. It's not phrased with any sort of pressure, which is extremely important, because if your goal on paper is to do one push-up, but your secret actual goal is 40 push-ups, your goal on paper doesn't matter. Now, you might have feelings of wanting to do more to feel accomplished. This is okay! That's exactly what this question addresses, giving you an opportunity to do more reps if you want *for any reason*.

There will be a time when "that's enough" is exactly what you need. There will be other times when "do I want to do more?" will be met with an emphatic "yes!" Give yourself credit, and the opportunity for more, and you'll do great things. This is a winning formula that satisfies the need for consistency and the desire to achieve more.

Remember: "That's a win. Do I want to do more?"

Tomorrow, we'll discuss the science of how exercise instantly improves nearly every one of your body's functions.

Day 24

Why Exercise Is a Panacea

"Yes, exercise is the catalyst. That's what makes everything happen: your digestion, your elimination, your sex life, your skin, hair, everything about you depends on circulation. And how do you increase circulation?"

~ Jack LaLanne

Today is special because I'll share my favorite exercise quote below. *Feel* this quote when you do your mini habit.

In his book *Brain Rules*, author John Medina explains why exercise is a panacea of sorts when it comes to feeling better and being healthier.

"When you exercise, you increase blood flow across the tissues of your body. This is because exercise stimulates the blood vessels to create a powerful, flow-regulating molecule called nitric oxide. As the flow improves, the body makes new blood vessels, which penetrate deeper and deeper into the tissues of the body. This allows more access to the bloodstream's goods and services, which include food distribution and waste disposal.

The more you exercise, the more tissues you can feed and the more toxic waste you can remove. This happens all over the body. That's why exercise improves the performance of most human functions."[1]

It's all about blood flow. Even five or ten seconds of flailing your limbs about will make a difference in how you feel. Try it now. Run in place aggressively for 10 seconds and *feel* what John Medina describes. How cool is that?

Part of changing your relationship with exercise is getting to know it in a different way. People often think of exercise as "that dreadful thing I must do to look better" or "because my doctor says so." How about instead of that: Exercise supercharges the blood flow in your body, making all of your systems work more efficiently! Even when moving isn't the most comfortable thing to do, this new understanding and perspective makes the effort feel worth it.

Tomorrow, we'll discuss something obvious that nobody does (because their daily goals are too big).

Day 25

Practice Winning

"Winning is a habit. Unfortunately, so is losing."

- Vince Lombardi

The best thing about easy wins is how stackable they are.

Reader Spotlight: "I have applied the principles in your mini habits book in the last 7 years and it has helped me achieve success in my surgical residency, my medical residency, my karate training, weekly tennis exercises, and also learning Hebrew."

You're here to practice winning. Many people don't practice winning and instead practice struggling to win occasionally while losing much of the time. Someone must have told us we must suffer to get results. This can't be further from the truth!

People at the highest level of their trade generally love it. Many of them *obsess* over even the most grueling work. To outsiders, that work may appear undesirable, but desires change as habits do. Many athletes, musicians, workers, fitness aficionados, and artists have fallen in love with the process.

Let's get excited about *winning*. There are habitual winners and losers. Here's how I differentiate the two. It's simple:

Loser: Plans X, Does Y

Winner: Plans X, Does X

Losers aren't losers in the derogatory sense of the word. There's nothing permanent about it. They can win just as easily! They simply mistake desire for ability. Let me give you a hypothetical example to explain.

Jacob desires to jump 40 feet in the air, but no human can do that. Thus, he loses every day. Jacob sighs and says, "Well, I guess I can't jump any higher." Nothing is wrong with Jacob, and he *can* train himself to jump higher than he currently does, but he won't get there by wishing to jump 40 feet. His desire causes him to accept total defeat instead of a small win that he can ultimately parlay into higher jumping ability.

Billions of people hold themselves back every day by demanding too much of themselves, falsely believing that the only height they can reach is the one they initially aim for.

Never forget this: It's better to win small than to lose big.

Never forget this: It's impossible to see your full potential early in your journey.

This is why big goals are the worst choice. They're supposed to be motivating, but they make it easier to lose AND they likely sell your potential short of what it can actually be. The only way to ensure winning forward progress *and* get closer to understanding your true potential is to continue to collect small wins every day.

There's one thing I discovered in my mini habit journey that blew my mind. And it sounds crazy to say it, but it is true in practice: when it comes to behavior change and momentum, small wins are just as impactful as big wins.

"I walk slowly, but I never walk backward."

~ Abraham Lincoln

Abraham Lincoln was born into poverty and ascended to become the President of the United States. His life was a true "zero to hero" story, and this quote was his formula. Forward motion is *everything*. And look at you! You've now moved forward 25 days in a row. I hope you can see today's message playing out in real time in your life.

Tomorrow poses an interesting question: Will you ever regret exercising? I use this question to this day to get myself moving.

Day 26

Regret Exercise?

"Remember, today is the tomorrow you worried about yesterday."

~ Dale Carnegie

Have you ever regretted exercising?

I ask myself this question frequently, because it comes in handy when I'm coming up with excuses not to work out.

Recently, I tweaked a muscle in my back while working out. It wasn't a serious injury, but it limited what I could do (as I didn't want to make it a serious injury). A few days later, I considered skipping the gym because my back wasn't 100%. But I knew I could exercise other areas carefully without risking further injury to it. Then I thought about this question, and the answer: I have never regretted exercising.

Even on the day that I injured my back, I still made progress and still felt good about my decision afterward. I understand that severe injuries are regrettable, but how remarkable that I didn't even regret that workout! One of my worst workouts turned out to be a net positive in my mind and most parts of my body.

People starting fresh need to know this: exercise feels better as you do it more. I can remember lifting weights when I was weaker, and the sensation was foreign and felt *extremely* annoying. Compare how you felt exercising on day one to now.

I'm no longer annoyed by lifting weights. In fact, during each set, I enjoy pushing myself. After each set, I love the feeling. After each workout, the "pump" feels incredible. Way before you become the Hulk, you get to feel like the Hulk.

Bottom line: Unless you hurt yourself from overexertion or poor form, you will never regret exercising.

Tomorrow, we talk about change and why it's so difficult to see as it happens.

Day 27

It's Hard to See Change

"The chains of habit are too weak to be felt until they are too strong to be broken."

- Samuel Johnson

Do your mini habit today. Trust this process.

When you change your life with new habits, it feels monumental, yet subtle. A decade ago, I didn't exercise consistently. Today, I love to exercise and do it daily. I've done it long enough to understand the full benefit on a conscious and subconscious level.

Looking back on how much I've changed and grown, the difference is astronomical. Baffling. But there's a reason why it also seems **so subtle**. Today, I'm living in accordance with my habits in the same way I always have. Objectively, it's a massive difference in behavior, but it doesn't feel that way because it's my new normal.

It's hard to think of a routine behavior as special, even if you're great at it. It's only when we consider who we once were that we realize just how special our normal has become. This is something you can look forward to.

To be succinct, it's hard to see change in (at least) two ways.

1. It's difficult to project how a change now may enable a

bigger change later. It's only when you ascend a mountain that you can even see what's on the other side of it. Don't assume the biggest change you can imagine today is your limit. You will see greater and greater possibilities as you progress.

2. When you change for real (brain change), you still live according to your preferences and abilities. Your preferences and abilities have changed, but you are still you. I don't try any harder today than I did when I didn't exercise. That's why I say sedentary living is almost never an effort problem. It's a behavior problem.

Tomorrow, we'll talk about why smoking is the golden standard for habits. I know that sounds strange, and I'm not advising you to light a cig, but you'll see what I mean.

Day 28

As Easy as Smoking

"Good habits, once established, are just as hard to break as are bad habits."

- Robert Puller

Have you done bonus reps recently? If not, do some today.

Have you ever thought about why it's so easy for people to get addicted to things? Smokers, for example, will tell you that it was easier to start smoking than it was to quit. But why is something like smoking a cigarette easier to make a habit than, say, going to the gym?

You could point to the nicotine or the feeling a person gets while smoking, sure. But exercise can provide a significant "high" as well (runner's high, pump from weights, etc.). There's a more important and more universal difference between the two. It's easier (and more accessible) to smoke a cigarette than to go to the gym. All you have to do is light it up and start smoking.

And this is perhaps the best explanation for why we're making our exercise habit "mini" in these 60 days.

Mini Habits for Fitness discarded slogan #420: "It's as easy as smoking!"

When it comes to forming good new habits, we can learn a lot from bad habits people pick up without trying. They tell us a lot about how our brain works and how to make behaviors more appealing. And, well, almost every bad habit people acquire begins by being **accessible and easy**.

"Just try it!" Jane said as she handed Nicole [any type of addictive substance]. And if Nicole wants to keep doing it, she can probably access it and use it daily. Let's make sure we do the same for fitness.

In truth, exercising has always been accessible and easy. You don't need any equipment because there are countless bodyweight exercises. There's no law that says you can't walk around or run in place as everyone else sits and waits (putting their metabolism to sleep).

Most people have developed a false notion of a "workout" being something they do in gym clothes for at least 20 minutes. That's patently false! You can exercise for 10 seconds in a banana costume at the mall. Studies have shown that exercise done in a banana costume counts double![1]

Tomorrow, we'll discuss exercise relationship issues that we're working to leave behind.

Day 29

Exercise Relationship Sourers to Drop

"Winning is only half of it. Having fun is the other half."

~ Bum Phillips

When in doubt, try a playful approach.

There are many reasons a person's relationship with exercise can sour. Often, those reasons are combined. We are working to leave these behind. Here are a few. See if you relate to these and if you can feel them slowly melting away with each successful mini habit win.

1. Pressure

Pressure from your doctor telling you to exercise and lose weight.
Pressure from your friends and family concerned for your health.
Pressure from yourself to look a certain way or improve your health.

2. Effort

The belief that exercise is a lot of effort with a questionable return.
Previous experiences of overexertion, which can do more harm

than good.
Previous experiences with intense workout programs that exhaust you.

3. Bad First Impressions

Exercise feels like punishment.
You've felt judged by others when exercising.
You've been injured from exercising.

4. Other Factors

You love to relax or play.
You don't enjoy exercise as much as doing other things.
You don't like feeling sweaty or dirty.

Whatever the factors, the end result is generally the same issue you find in human relationships--**resentment**. You can grow to resent a behavior, whether or not it is the behavior's fault. It's mostly circumstantial and situational and is fixed by experiencing the same behavior in a new way, like we're doing now.

Exercise is rewarding. It can be fun. It can be low-pressure. It can be about *you* and *what you want* instead of anyone else's influence. Best of all, it can be better-than-easy.

If we don't enjoy something, we want it to at least be easy (for me, that's washing the dishes: I love my dishwasher!). Exercise is something that provides significant internal and external rewards, meaning we can grow to enjoy the challenge of it. Your exercise mini habit is easy now without the relational baggage, but later you won't mind a long run or a tough weightlifting session. You'll crave them!

Tomorrow, we're going to talk about something that annoys me more than words can express. People are obsessed with doing

30 days of something. Thirty days is not a magical amount of time for behavior change. Sixty days is only slightly magical.

Day 30

Does it Flip the Switch?

"Habits are safer than rules; you don't have to watch them. And you don't have to keep them, either. They keep you."

- Frank Crane

Do your mini habit today, or you'll turn back into a pumpkin (according to some).

We've reached the magical Day 30. This is the day in which all of your dreams come true and you never have to work another day in your life. Why else would half of self-help books be 30 days to this, 30 days to that?

Day 30 is no different than Day 29 or Day 31.

People decide to assign significance to random numbers for marketing purposes. You could say the same about this book's "60 days." One difference, however, is that 60 days is *very* close to the 2009 study that found habits formed in an average of 66 days.

Given these are mini habits (easy), and that difficulty plays a role in how quickly habits develop, it figures that 60 days is plenty of time to form a habit. It's a nice, clean two months of time, but it's also enough to provide a habitual foundation (30 days is very iffy in that regard).

If you're able to absorb the spirit of this method into your psyche, you will learn to look at processes of your chosen systems instead of goals or milestones. Milestones are points in time, but processes are lasting and repeatable. Processes generate milestones without even trying!

Do you want to pat yourself on the back for making it 30 days? No problem, I raise my glass to you. But you know what's better? Celebrate completing your mini habit *today*. Celebrate 30 *individual* wins instead of one arbitrary milestone. That's 30x more celebrations! We aim to master the day because that's the structure of a human's existence--your life is one giant string of days. Sleep cycles and routines make the 24-hour day the ideal focal point for change.

Success is one small action at a time and one day at a time. Milestones are fine, and you can celebrate them, but don't ever mistake them as being the goal or prize.

Are you ready to climb higher? See you tomorrow in a brand new section!

Part II

A New Relationship with Exercise

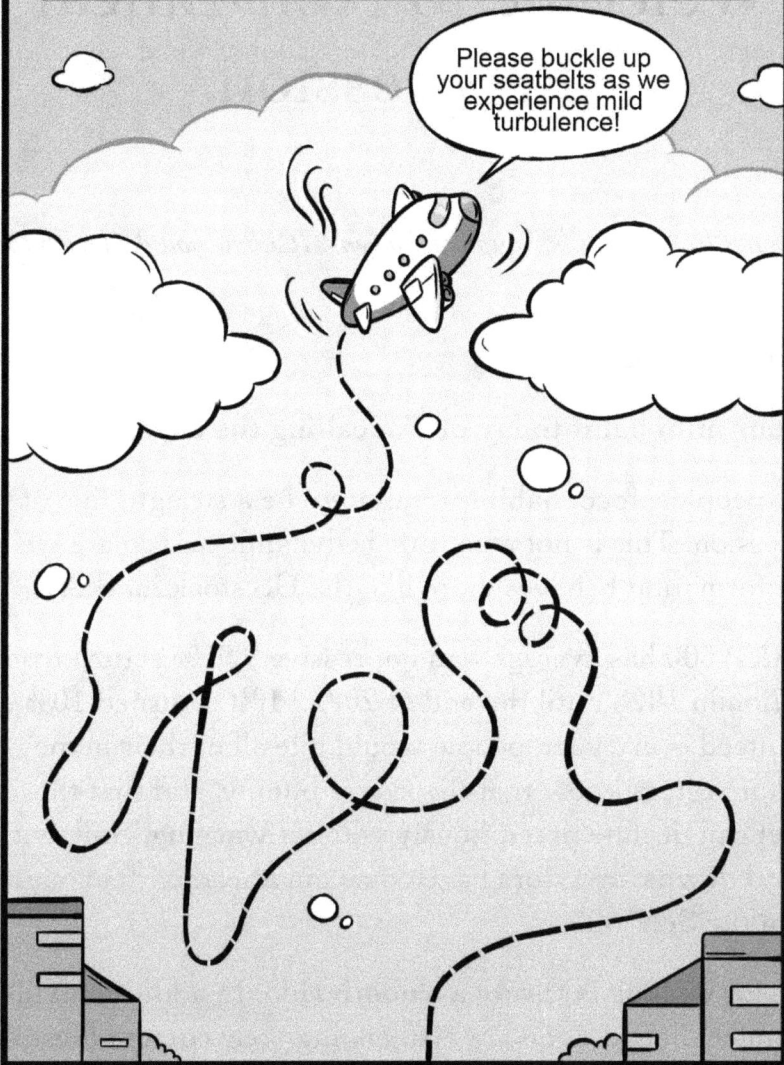

Day 31

Welcome to Non-Linear Progression

"Life is not linear; you have ups and downs. It's how you deal with the troughs that defines you."

~ Michael Lee-Chin

Do your mini habit today or I'm calling the cops.

Many people expect habit formation to be a straight line of progression. This is not true. Life is dynamic and so are we. Habit formation behaves more like the US stock market.

The S&P 500 has averaged an impressive 9.95% return from its inception in 1928 until the end of 2023.[1] If it returned 10% guaranteed every year, people would pile all of their money into it. But investors know that the ride is bumpy, and that the market can decline precipitously without warning. Still, with the ups and downs, investors have come out ahead with enough time in the S&P 500.

Behavior change is rarely a smooth ride. In addition to life's random challenges, you are challenging your current lifestyle, stretching the limits of your comfort zone. With a behavior this small and easy, it's not *much* of a stretch, but it is still less comfortable than the norm, and that matters.

Just because your behavior is small does not change the fact that you will have good days and bad days. Your mini habit will help you win on bad days, the ones that kill regular goals. If you can succeed in the widest variety of moods and situations, you will have massive success.

We're shooting for higher highs and higher lows over time.

By the way, if you're ever curious to know what's habitual and what's not, pay attention to your inner dialogue. Your habits are like hired lobbyists in your brain, constantly persuading you to do them. Non-habits are often the opposite, requiring effort to even consider doing them.

Your exercise mini habit is so small you can force it for now. Later, exercise will be the thing you think of often and want to do.

Tomorrow I'll answer a question you might have: How does the transition from small (mini) to big actually work?

Day 32

How Small Habits Become Big Habits

"Consistency of performance is essential. You don't have to be exceptional every week but as a minimum you need to be at a level that even on a bad day you get points on the board."

~ Sean Dyche (English football manager)

A subpar performance on a bad day is one of the finest wins you'll ever experience with exercise. Because it isn't a zero.

Small habits become big habits by establishing a firm floor and then raising it.

A regular goal aims for a ceiling and allows you to fall through the floor. Whoops. It feels good when you hit the upper target, but when you don't, you fall through the floor into an endless abyss of failure. Okay, I'm being dramatic, but the point is that all-or-nothing behaviors don't enable you to *build from the bottom up*.

All stable structures are built from the bottom up.

I worked construction one summer, and I noticed we never built the roof first. There's something logical about making sure your current foundation can support each structure you add on top of it, right? Building a new behavior in your life works very well this way. Small habits give you familiarity, and that's the foundation for big success.

Your subconscious brain builds a friendly relationship with the behaviors you repeat the most. If you can do something every day, your brain will learn to tolerate it (at a minimum) because of familiarity. This is largely a business decision at first. The brain goes like, "If we're gonna be doing this every day, I don't want to have to expend a lot of energy thinking about it. Let me automate this process."

If you've already heard me say this or find this book **repetitive**, there's a reason for that...

I want you to be very familiar with the power of familiarity!

Some people may "hate" their job, but they still come in and know what to expect from it. Whether it's a bad job or relationship, **familiarity** can keep people around a lot longer than is ideal. And what about all of those dumb advertisements on TV? You think they don't know how annoying they are? They know, but they also don't care because it gets their brand *seen* and familiarized.

Familiarity is power, but here's the thing: Exercise isn't like a bad job (or a lame commercial). It's more like a best friend-- you'll love it as you get to know it without the baggage. We're getting familiar with exercise in a healthy way.

The downside of exercise? It takes effort. That's it. Benefits? Too many to list, but here are some broad *categories* of benefits...

- Improved physical health
- Improved mental health
- Improved emotional control
- More energy
- More confidence
- More attractive physique

- Longer lifespan
- Increased quality of life
- Increased strength

Within each of those are specific benefits. For example, as regards physical health, exercise improves blood flow to every organ in your body. It strengthens your heart, and it decreases your risk for most diseases.

How is *this* the thing that people don't like doing? How is *this* the thing that we sometimes feel is a chore instead of an opportunity and gift? Many people are just not familiar enough with it and those insane benefits! They may have seen a toxic and broken version of it instead and avoided it.

Now that your habit is taking shape, tomorrow I'm going to poke holes in it. For better or worse, we must respect that behavior change can always happen, meaning no habit is invincible.

Day 33

Habits Are not Invincible

"Your body is malleable; you can sculpt it over time with daily habits of diet and exercise. The law of accommodation reminds us that the body may change slowly, but it will change."

~ Dan Millman

After 33 consecutive mini wins, your body might look the same, but your brain doesn't.

Our bodies are malleable, as are the habits that shape them. Habits are comparatively the strongest and most resilient behaviors, but even they can be weakened intentionally or unintentionally. This is good news, because otherwise our bad habits would drive us into the ground with no recourse. But it's important to recognize this fact with good habits.

I get the sense that modern culture has made habits appear failproof. If you just form the habit, you'll never struggle again! In some ways, that can be true, but it isn't completely accurate.

If you form a strong exercise habit, you are more likely to stick with it than stop it. But if your situation suddenly changes, it can jeopardize that. The most common reverse card in our case is illness or injury. Getting sick or hurt could make it difficult or even unwise to exercise, and in that time, your exercise habit will weaken.

Two of the worst exercise slumps in my life happened after I got

COVID-19. I had milder cases and was only down about a week each time, but it also took a toll on my energy levels in the following weeks and interrupted my exercise routines. But there is hope! It was actually this experience that helped me see the biggest benefit of habits.

While my exercise habit was not invincible--I stopped during illness and even for some time after it--I was able to restart it without issue. When you reactivate a dormant habit, those neural pathways spring back to life, and you can be right back to where you were (or close to it). This makes addictions dangerous, as one relapse can lead to a total collapse. But it's also why good habits are so valuable to develop.

Remember this: Habits are not invincible, but they enable long stretches of success and can be restarted at will if something interrupts your progress. As your exercise habit grows in strength, you'll find yourself figuring out how to (smartly and carefully) exercise around minor injuries that would once serve as an excuse to rest. You'll find yourself easily able to bounce back if you stop for a time for whatever reason.

Tomorrow, let's talk about a different kind of reward you can expect with your developing habit.

Day 34

A Different Kind of Rewarding

"Enjoy the satisfaction that comes from doing little things well."

~ H. Jackson Brown, Jr.

Make this current streak the best exercise streak you've ever had.

Habit formation is exciting, but not in the way an event is exciting. This won't feel like the rush you get from a concert, an epiphany, or any one-time experience.

Foundational good habits provide a deep and long-lasting reward. It's a constant, subtle sense of joy that you are living in precisely the way you intend. This clarification is important.

Before a behavior is habit, you might treat it as a celebratory event. I did. **Before exercise was a habit, I would feel an *enormous* sense of accomplishment after working out.** It seems like a good thing, but all it meant was that my behavior was *enormously* far from habit.

Observe how you feel after doing your mini habit (and bonus reps if desired) today. With such small habits, you may not feel a big sense of accomplishment, but *that's okay*, because this aligns with how you'll feel as the habit grows bigger and stronger.

We can find joy in doing *something better than zero*. The cumulative effect of so many non-zero days strung together feels amazing. It's a powerful feeling to go from intermittent success to winning every day.

There are a few choices you make regularly that show if your relationship with exercise is healthy or needs work. Let's see where you are tomorrow.

Day 35

I Can Tell with One Question

"Everywhere is within walking distance if you have the time."

~ Steven Wright

If you want a challenge, do 10+ minutes of exercise today. If not, just do the mini habit and I'll still shake your hand.

A good test of your relationship with exercise is your default choice in the following situations...

Escalator or stairs?

Any open parking spot or circle 44 times to find the closest spot?

Drive somewhere close or walk or bike?

Use the moving walkway or not?

If you *always* find yourself seeking the more convenient option, it's because you don't prefer moving or, perhaps more accurately, you don't *think* you like moving. Or perhaps it's because everyone else lines up at the escalator as the stairs are empty so it seems "correct." In any case, the more active choice is always better for you. It immediately increases blood flow throughout your body and provides health benefits for free.

Dani Blum nicely summarized an eye-opening recent study[1] in her NY Times article[2]: "Those who engaged in one or two-minute bursts of exercise roughly three times a day, like speed-walking while commuting to work or rapidly climbing stairs, showed a nearly 50 percent reduction in cardiovascular mortality risk and a roughly 40 percent reduction in the risk of dying from cancer as well as all causes of mortality, compared with those who did no vigorous spurts of fitness."

If you were given the same options again but taking the stairs came with a 50% reduction in cardiovascular mortality risk (exactly what the study showed for similar activities), who *wouldn't* take the stairs? I'm glad we're finally seeing some studies come out on these smaller decisions we make, because too many people believe that these decisions don't matter.

Every step counts. Every choice counts. You can make a *massive* difference in your life by making just slightly better choices than you used to in these situations.

Modern society has trained us to avoid stairs when there's an escalator. If you're able to take the stairs, I encourage you to take them! It is always worth it. It makes me a little bit sad when I see people lining up at the escalator and I'm the only person on the stairs. I try to take the stairs at least half of the time (escalators are fun so I can't go 100%). I hope to see you on the stairs!

The next time you see an escalator, a small Stephen may appear on your shoulder (angel) and say, "Why not take the stairs?"

Tomorrow, we discuss momentum, the most powerful force in personal growth!

Day 36

Momentum Is the Way

"The world is wide, and I will not waste my life in friction when it could be turned into momentum."

~ Frances E. Willard

You're not merely building a powerful habit, you're creating positive momentum every day. Note how your physical feelings and thoughts change the second you engage in exercise. You become *active*.

Mini habits provide a path to habit formation--the obvious main benefit. But the secondary benefit is nearly as good--daily momentum creation.

Momentum is a wonder. My last book was called *The Magic of Momentum* for a reason, and it wasn't marketability. Don't feel like doing something? Start anyway and watch what happens. Most of the time, you'll feel a shift and warm up to the activity. In exercise, you literally warm up once your blood gets pumping!

I want you to experience and embrace the joy of the present moment. Your mini habit will open the door to that. Instead of being bogged down by doubts about what you think you can't do or overwhelmed about how far you feel you need to go, you can jump in and let momentum carry you to a great workout.

I have had the intention of writing 50 words or doing one push-up thousands of times (my mini habits). I've exceeded those intentions thousands of times because of momentum. You don't need big goals to get big short-term results!

What I'm telling you works, but you have to buy in.

Get started before you feel confident. Jump in without expectations. Now you're in motion, and momentum will bring you closer to the results you want.

Tomorrow, I want to congratulate you. Show up and be showered with praise!

Day 37

You Exercise Every Day

"Good habits are worth being fanatical about."

~ John Irving

During your mini habit today, internalize this: "I exercise every day now." This can be part of your identity.

Reader Spotlight: "My expectations were drowning me, and my mini habits pulled me up to the surface."

We are 37 days in, and here's something amazing. You can say that you exercise every day. That sounds impressive and is a powerful new identity trait to have.

This is not a "gimmick" because the behaviors are small. This is *world-class consistency*, which is exactly what creates world-class people. Daily exercise is the same platform upon which world-class athletes have built their bodies and abilities. They train every day. So do you.

Now, you may or may not have the athletic ceiling of an Olympian, but your physical potential should not be a factor in whether or not exercise is "right for you." I see too many people (my past self included) look at their current state or genetics and think they're too far from the perfect human genetics to bother trying. Why try if you can't ever reach the top? Here are a few reasons...

1. Because exercise is integral to improving and maintaining health, and we all desire good health!

2. You can strive to be the best version of yourself. It's cliché and cheesy, but think about what that really means--a future version of you that can totally outclass the current version of you. That's exciting and interesting to think about.

3. Forget about your body shape and physical abilities for a moment. Internal change is the best change you're going to experience: improved blood flow, healthier organs, better digestion, increased confidence, improved mood, and so much more.

4. You will grow. The worst feeling in life is stagnation or the thought that you have nothing going for you and aren't making progress. Exercise is a guaranteed way to grow stronger every day. It is the easy choice when you don't know what else to do with your life.

5. Unbelievably valuable ancillary benefits await you: improved sleep, libido, energy, endurance, and reduced pain (pain often comes from muscle weakness and/or imbalance) are a few known benefits of exercise.

All of this is yours to have. The only requirement is a dedication to move and use your body, which comes easier and easier as you learn to enjoy it.

Tomorrow, we'll dig into the details of this book's subtitle. What does the path to "loving" exercise look like?

Day 38

Tolerate, Like, Love

"If you change the way you look at things, the things you look at change."

~ Wayne Dyer

Today's Task: Do your mini habit today. I think I may have said this before. But it remains just as important as day one!

The general progression of a typical exercise relationship goes like this:

1. Hate it
2. Annoyed by it
3. Tolerate it
4. Neutral
5. Slightly enjoy it
6. Like it
7. Love it

If you started out hating exercise, you might not get to the "love it" stage in these 60 days. That's okay! Any progress or "upgrade" in this list represents a massive decrease in resistance to the behavior. I don't want you to get discouraged if you aren't obsessed and in love with exercise yet, because more than likely, you have already made a meaningful move from where you began.

I used to hate mushrooms. I wouldn't eat them. Today, I tolerate some mushrooms in some dishes, which expands my dietary options. The more you learn to love exercise, the more types you'll be willing to try/do and the longer you'll be willing to work out.

These days, I will even walk on the treadmill even though I have never liked doing that. I really enjoy exercise in general and feel good about doing it, so even treadmills (my exercise mushrooms) are no problem.

At the end of the book, you can take another fitness relationship assessment to see how much you've changed. Learning to tolerate exercise for some people will be a massive victory. If you hated exercising, tolerating it completely changes the game. You can do something that you tolerate a lot easier than something you hate, and those increased opportunities will help you continue to improve the relationship.

Very few who experience the full effects of exercise are able to resist it. Many people simply never get to that point because the road to get there is littered with shame, pressure, and extremes.

Tomorrow, we're going to talk about something you may be familiar with by now.

Day 39

Familiarity Is Everything

"A reliable way to make people believe in falsehoods is frequent repetition, because familiarity is not easily distinguished from truth. Authoritarian institutions and marketers have always known this fact."

~ Daniel Kahneman

Do your mini habit even if it's Monday! This has a 14.28% chance of being relevant.

Familiarity underlies all habitual behavior; it is safety, comfort, and truth. Familiarity is also extremely dangerous to the mind, as Kahneman points out here. Because we rely on familiarity so much, we can easily mistake it for truth. When you don't exercise for an extended period of time or do it intermittently, you get familiar with *that* lifestyle. You may begin to believe the following things without realizing it.

1. I'm okay without exercising.
2. It's fine to not move much throughout the day.
3. Exercise isn't important to me.
4. I couldn't get in decent shape even if I tried.

Those are lies. They are dangerous lies, born from familiarity with a sedentary lifestyle that can be mistaken for truth. All of these potential beliefs should easily be proven false by now. You've been exercising daily for 39 days. You can feel it, can't you? It's *much better* to get that extra movement in, even in mini doses. Exercise becomes extremely important to everyone the moment they understand (through experience) its benefits. There are even more significant benefits waiting for you later in this journey.

Over this past month or so, you've gotten more familiar with your chosen form of exercise as well as the practice of exercising daily. That familiarity is critical. You're giving exercise a chance to compete with any existing familiarity you may have with sedentary living. I have a lot of familiarity with sedentary living and exercise. Being familiar with both, I choose exercise often because it's easy to do now and I know it's better.

Tomorrow, we clarify something that may surprise you in a fitness book--sedentary habits aren't 100% bad.

Day 40

Sedentary Habits Aren't All Bad

"Rest when you're weary. Refresh and renew yourself, your body, your mind, your spirit. Then get back to work."

~ Ralph Marston

I'm proud of you. Victory today marks 40 straight wins.

As I write this, even with a strong exercise habit, I am still sedentary at times. I've had my sedentary habit for a very long time, longer than my exercise habit.

Some may see sedentary living as a void or blank space that can be filled in with other activities, but it's actually a conditioned behavior. It's important to see it this way because otherwise you may underestimate its "pull" on you. You need to create opposing habits to compete with it.

But let's not go overboard here. We're not out to eliminate rest, we're here to achieve a greater balance. We need to move *and* rest. Sitting is not the enemy![1] Recovery is prioritized among athletes for good reason--that's when their hard work actually takes effect. Weightlifting, for example, creates tiny tears in the muscle, which are then rebuilt bigger and stronger *during periods of rest.*

People who love working out tend to also love relaxation. They go together! Kicking your feet up on the couch is an excellent reward for a workout. And while we're not always doing full workouts in these 60 days of mini habits, we can still practice the beautiful synergy of exertion and rest.

If you have sedentary habits, remember that shame regarding them is not going to help you improve them. Shame is never the way forward. Instead, keep up your fitness mini habit and continue to cultivate a better relationship with exercise. This exercise habit is going to be a fun alternative to some of the sedentary habits you might currently have. One of the best things about exercising is that it makes rest more rewarding.

Bottom line: To celebrate movement is not to demonize rest. Movement and rest complement each other. The ratio of movement to rest is key for health and happiness, but that ideal will differ for each person.

In the next section, we'll talk about the fundamentals and how to make exercise more enjoyable. This becomes increasingly important as you take on greater fitness challenges in the future.

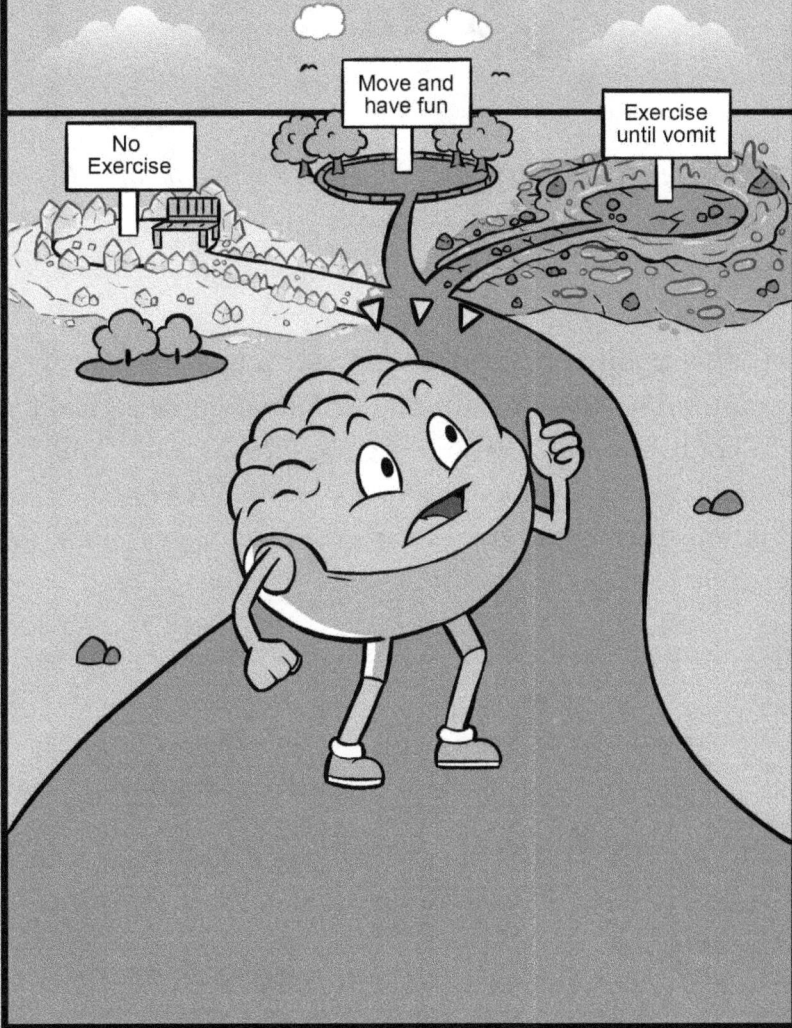

Day 41

Is Exercise Miserable or Fun?

"I'm not trying to be sexy. It's just my way of expressing myself when I move around."

~ Elvis Presley

Day 41 Checkpoint: Nice job. You've reached the last checkpoint before the end. If you are fully confident, feel free to increase your mini habit requirement *a little bit more*. This is not a call to make your mini habit a mega habit. We're still building a foundation. Respect that and the progress you've made to find a sweet spot.

Example: You started with one push-up a day. On the Day 21 checkpoint, you doubled it to two. Today, you might raise it to five. (We can double or even triple our mini habit target as we progress because it's that easy. It's our floor, not our ceiling.)

Make sure that your new target reflects a challenge that is as easy for you as Day 1 was. You may also keep your mini habit the same.

In these next 10 days, we're going to be discussing the fundamentals of exercise and habits. They're not always so obvious, such as this first one.

Exercise should be fun and enjoyable whenever possible.

This is so critical, and I believe that many people miss the mark here. You don't have to be miserable as you learn to love fitness. You can and should make it fun.

I live in Florida and today was a high of 99 degrees. I went outside and played basketball for 45 minutes. It was brutal heat, but I loved it.

If I were merely shooting hoops, I might get bored or decide that it's too hot to bother with it. But I came up with a fun shooting challenge. I often listen to music while I play, and, randomly, when a song came on, I decided to shoot from five spots on the court, progressing to a more difficult shot after I made each one. If I miss, I must rebound and try the spot again until I make it. The first shot is a layup. The fifth and final shot of the round is a very long three-pointer.

I ended up completing four rounds of five shots made before the song ended. And a shooting challenge was born![1]

Here's the thing: Not only is this challenge more fun than just shooting hoops, it's also a much better workout. If I fail, my competitive nature kicks in and I push myself to try again. I want to win!

This shooting game translates into a HIIT workout. These workouts are denoted by short but very intense periods of exercise followed by rest. They've been shown to have similar health benefits as moderate-intensity exercise, but they take far less time.[2] HIIT has also been shown to be effective for fat loss.[3]

While I started out at the gym "just showing up" (perfectly fine), now I track my workouts and try to beat my previous lifts in weight or reps. It's fun and challenging and also more effective for muscle growth. I use an app called "Hevy" and highly recommend it for iPhone and Android users (it's free as of writing).

For every piece of advice on proper form or what exercise to do, there should be five pieces of information about how to make it more fun. The more enjoyable your experience, the more you'll do it and the faster your brain will make that behavior a habit. Tomorrow, I'm going to give you four of my favorite ideas to make exercise more fun.

Day 42

Fundamentals of Fun

"Just play. Have fun. Enjoy the game."

~ Michael Jordan

These fun tips can help you do bonus reps today!

Creativity is paramount for making exercise fun, but there are a few principles that tend to work best.

The number one fun factor for exercise is competition.

Sports are so much fun that billions of people watch other people play them! The heart of sport is competition. When I'm playing full-court basketball, I'm trying to win, not looking at the clock or thinking about the calories I've burned.

But when it comes to exercise, not everyone has the access or ability to play sports. That's okay because your main competitor can be yourself and the challenges you give yourself.

- Try to beat your previous best time.
- Challenge yourself to complete a certain number of reps.

Some people aren't as competitive as others, and that's fine. There are more options for you coming up!

Music can elevate most exercise experiences.

Yesterday I explained my basketball shooting challenge. It's for the duration of one song, which is a lot more fun than a clock (though that would work too). I highly recommend creating a challenge based on the duration of a song you like. Dance all out for its duration, or create a more specific challenge.

Many gymgoers bring headphones, but I also enjoy going to the gym without music. Do what works for you.

Incentivize, Incentivize, Incentivize

Bribery still exists for a reason. When people have a greater incentive to do something, they are more likely to do it! Best of all, it's completely legal to bribe yourself to exercise.

At one point in my life, I created a points system in which I earned points through exercise and could "spend" those points on things like going to a movie or getting a new video game. The reason this book is not a point-system book? It didn't work, as it wasn't designed for *consistency* like a mini habit is. Still, concepts like this can certainly be implemented to varying degrees once your exercise habit has a stronger foundation.

To this day, I will bribe myself. I don't like leg day, so I may tell myself, "Do legs today, and you'll earn a movie ticket."

Gamification of Your Workout

It's easy to gamify your workout. Buy yourself some dice or take them from that one board game you never play. Roll the dice and pay the price! Some options:

- Number rolled = type of exercise (push-ups, pull-ups, lunges, bodyweight squats)
- Number rolled = number of reps (1-6 with one die or 2-12 with two dice)
- Number rolled = package deal (i.e., rolling a four means you

have to do 8 push-ups, rolling a nine means you have to do 15 sit-ups)

You can add all sorts of fun wrinkles. Maybe one number represents a prize or treat not related to exercise. Roll a 12, get a small piece of chocolate! Rule of thumb: If it helps get you interested and engaged in doing physical activity, it's a good thing.

Tomorrow's topic is the one nobody expected. There's a significant benefit to being out of shape when it comes to exercising.

Day 43

The Advantage of Being out of Shape

"If all you can do is crawl, then start crawling."

~ Rumi

Aim to master exercise psychology. You're not "struggling" because you're out of shape--you're burning more fat than if you were in perfect shape, and you *feel that intensity*. Now the exercise feels better and more productive. Try it today. As you exercise, notice how your psychology changes the way you perceive and feel exercise. (Note: this is also how I enjoy the taste of kale now. Trained associations can change how you feel.)

Something weird happened early on in my one push-up challenge. Prior to doing one push-up or more per day, I hadn't been actively exercising. And I noticed, within the first few days, I actually felt a little bit stronger from very few push-ups and very little time spent working out.

There's a phrase in the weightlifting world known as "newbie gains."

The more out of shape you are, the more exercise will positively impact your body. New lifters gain more muscle mass than experienced bodybuilders. The more fat you carry,

the more (and faster) you'll lose with exercise.

That is a fact, and it works perfectly with the progression of someone going from inactive to active. At first, exercise feels toughest because of mental resistance and physical weakness, but it also gives you the best physical results. The more body fat you have, the more you'll lose (and the faster you'll lose it) with exercise. The less muscle you have, the more and faster you'll gain it with strength training (relatively speaking).

As your fitness progresses, *it requires relatively more work to get equivalent results*. This is bad news if your habit can't support it. That's why a gradual approach works so well--higher difficulty is balanced by your increased reliability and fitness level.

"Get fit slow" is a tough sell in the marketplace, but for the few who aren't snared by the grifters promising fast results, it's a blessing to have something real that you can build upon for the rest of your life. Weight loss shows make people throw up from pushing their body too hard. How are we supposed to want to exercise if it makes us throw up?

This is not to say that get-fit-fast methods can't ever work. It's simply to say that they're not *designed* to work long-term for most people. They're designed to attract people. You could say that they attract 95% of people and work for 5% of people. This book aims to work for 95% of people. It may only attract a small percentage of people, but I hope those who try it tell others about it.

Another issue with intense exercise programs is how intimidating they can be. Exercise can be challenging, but it should never *intimidate* you. Exercise is simple. Let's talk about that tomorrow.

Day 44

Exercise Is Simple

"If you're flammable and have legs, you are never blocking a fire exit."

~ Mitch Hedberg

Do your mini habit today. You're good at this now!

Reader Spotlight: "Mini habits I can handle, even at my advanced age of 75!"

The fundamental component of exercise is movement. And instead of harping on about the many incredible benefits of exercise, let's take a look at the other side to gain some perspective about how physically easy and simple it is. Let's visualize what it means to be sedentary, which is defined by a lack of movement.

If you think about it, your body kind of works like a factory. Your heart is pumping blood, moving it constantly throughout your body. That blood transports vital things (i.e., oxygen) to vital places (i.e., the brain). Cells repair organs. Organs cleanse out toxins. Special cells fight invaders. Malfunctioning cells get terminated and replaced with healthy cells.

When your "body factory" is stagnant from lack of movement, it becomes dysfunctional. Things happen later, less effectively, and/or less efficiently. But the moment you start to move, even a little bit, everything comes to life. Your heart pumps harder and blood flow increases. That means more cells can repair and get repaired, organs do their jobs better, micronutrients are distributed where they're needed faster, and even your bowels move better (walking after meals is a great idea!).

I used to think of exercise in less sophisticated terms, like lifting weights makes you stronger, or running makes you leaner. But I think the more nuanced science of movement is far more compelling and interesting. When you move, you improve your body at the cellular level, and you don't have to wait for it to happen. It begins the moment you start to move.

It's no wonder that I always feel better after a workout. My body is literally an upgraded version of what it was prior to moving. This perspective can really help you if you feel you have a "long way to go" to reach your fitness goals, such as if you have a lot of weight to lose. To lose weight the right way takes time, but you don't have to wait at all to experience these immediate and rewarding benefits of vascular flow. You'll feel it right away.

The next time you find yourself feeling lazy, remember this, and imagine your body's factory at a standstill. All you have to do is get up and move in some way, and you'll come to life internally.

We've already done this once, but try it again; I want you to experience it at least twice in these 60 days (apart from your mini habit) *while observing your body*. It'll be easy and interesting.

Before you start, take note of how you feel. Your circulation, your mind, your energy level, your mood. Got it? Okay, now try this.

Get up and dance hard, do push-ups, or run in place for **just 30 seconds**. If you're in a wheelchair, try shadowboxing for 30 seconds. Move!

Done? Now take note of any physiological changes you feel

compared to 30 seconds ago. Observe your...

- ✓ Heart: pumping.
- ✓ Blood: moving.
- ✓ Body: warmer.
- ✓ Mind: sharper.
- ✓ Energy: increased.
- ✓ Cells: activated.
- ✓ Mood: improved.
- ✓ Status: active.

That's a BIG return on your 30-second investment, no? And you have this power available to you at all times. Don't let limited thinking like "only a 30-minute workout is worthwhile" deprive you of this gift ever again! You just proved you can achieve a significant biological change across your entire body in 30 seconds.

That just shows how simple and easy it is to exercise. It's movement. The results are anything but simple--they're a robust and complex marvel of cellular rejuvenation!

But what exercise is best? Good question. See you tomorrow.

Day 45

The Best Exercise

"Walking is the best possible exercise. Habituate yourself to walk very far."

~ Thomas Jefferson

Do some bonus reps if you haven't lately. Going through the motions can work, but for best results we must connect our fitness desires to our actions. The mini habit sparks us to move closer to where we want to be.

When people ask about the best exercise, the automatic answer is "the kind that you'll do." Certainly, that is impossible to argue with, because we need to move, and so whatever makes us most eager to move is the most valuable. But beyond that, I have real interest in the actual question. If pitted against every other form of exercise, what is the overall best choice?

The comparative factors are so numerous it seems impossible to separate them--calorie burn rate, enjoyment factor, functionality benefits, strength, endurance, longevity, injury risk, flexibility, time to recover, ease of access, weight loss, and so on. How can one possibly be crowned as best?

Well, I'm crowning one here, and I'll explain why. It's walking. For starters, walking is the most functionally important form of exercise for humankind. And it's no coincidence that it also happens to have some of the greatest benefits. For those who are able, walking is our primary form of transportation. We should get used to it and get good at it!

Walking is also special because it is truly a sweet spot for exercise. Let me elaborate.

Typing on my keyboard now is technically movement and takes some energy, but it isn't enough to raise my heart rate. It has very little impact on me physically. *It isn't enough to move the needle.*

High-intensity exercise is great, but it comes with drawbacks. For example, intense exercise burns a lot of calories, but it also makes you want to eat more calories. Plus, it requires recovery time, in which you may be less active than usual. *It can be too much to handle.*

Walking is a low-intensity exercise, yet it burns lots of calories. Not only that, studies have found that walking does not increase appetite to the same degree as higher-intensity exercise (a massive benefit if weight loss is your goal).[1] Walking is enough exercise to matter, but not too much to handle.

As for recovery, I've been sore after some days of walking 25,000+ steps. But even then, I could still walk the next day. And, like all forms of exercise, the more you walk, the better conditioned you'll be to walk more. Some of my trips to Europe have resulted in several days in a row with a very high step count. I noticed that I slept very well those nights despite being in a noisy hostel.

If you want to make walking more like a workout, you can simply increase your walking speed or go hiking (to add incline). Walking is so fundamental to our experience and has unique benefits for getting fit that I can't imagine anything else being better. It's the perfect way to introduce more movement into your life.

While I would say that walking is the best overall and most fundamental human exercise, I still have to admit the truth of the cliché mentioned earlier: "The best exercise is the one you'll do." Whatever you enjoy most, absolutely do that. The idea isn't to exercise so that you don't need to exercise anymore, it's to make exercise an enjoyable, integral, and positive part of your life.

Tomorrow, we talk about an unfortunate truth--humans will always underestimate the power of small steps. It's hardwired into us.

Day 46

Why You Will Always Underestimate Small Steps

"Small opportunities are often the beginning of great enterprises."

~ Demosthenes

Skip today, it doesn't really matter much. Just kidding! Every day is a small part of a greater foundation that you're building. Keep it up.

I've written five books about small steps, *using small steps* over a decade of my life. I popularized the concept in 2013 with the original *Mini Habits* book. The *Mini Habits* strategy changed my life in several areas. Most notably, it changed my relationship with fitness and writing itself. I also use the strategy in everyday life to do things like laundry, the dishes, or getting my fence fixed.

And yet... I continue to underestimate small steps. *Me!* Often. I know if I can still underestimate small steps after being immersed in them for a decade, everyone does it. Of all people, I would be the person to have learned not to underestimate them anymore!

In real, practical terms, this means I often have to force myself to "show up, do something small, and see what happens." It's as if I haven't seen it *thousands of times* successfully play out. But that's something I want to clarify: Because I have seen it play out, I'm better able to force myself to do it now.

Even though I love to exercise now and I seek it out, that hasn't changed the fact that it takes significant effort. It's rarely the path of least resistance to drive to the gym and work out for an hour. I do it because I enjoy it. But some days are more challenging and tiring than others, and that's when I can rely on "just show up and give it a shot."

Habits have become so mainstream and popular today, I worry that they've been built up into more than they actually are. The primary benefit of a good fitness habit is a *healthy relationship with movement/exercise and decreased resistance to action.* You'll still have bad days. You'll still find it challenging at times. But it will be much easier overall to:

A. get yourself to exercise
B. perform the exercise(s) in increasingly greater quantity/ intensity
C. enjoy the entire process

Before it's habitual, it's so much effort just to muster the strength *to make the decision to exercise.* Then you have to exert yourself on top of that. It isn't easy at first, unless you make it a miniature, easy version to start. That's what we're doing.

You've undoubtedly had some success already--maybe you've gone above and beyond a few days with bonus reps just because you started. But, even with these experiences, it's normal to still underestimate the power of small steps.

You've seen the power of getting started with a small goal with low or no expectations. Remind yourself of this power as often as you can. If you continue to show up every day, you will succeed.

Show up, get started, and let momentum help you.

I used to believe I needed more motivation. But that doesn't make sense, does it? I didn't want it enough? Really? Did I need a gun to my head to get in shape? No, this is just an excuse for the worst and most often repeated strategy for fitness. Tomorrow, we'll break up with motivational reliance for good.

Day 47

Waves of Motivation

"Hope begins in the dark, the stubborn hope that if you just show up and try to do the right thing, the dawn will come. You wait and watch and work: you don't give up."

~ Anne Lamott

Exercise isn't always something you feel like doing, even after establishing a strong habit. The reps you put in today are training you to show up in all situations because you know the reward is worth it.

It's day 47. What if you *still* don't always feel like doing your mini habit? It's so small and easy, and should be close to habit by now. What gives?

The fundamental truth about human motivation is that it comes and goes. Waves of motivation can be strong enough to override established habits. But in low tide, when there's no motivation, only habits remain.

Think about this scenario: any time a person gets "sick and tired of being sick and tired" and marches to the gym in determination, their motivational wave has overridden their sedentary lifestyle preferences (i.e., habits). Great! Until a week later, when the same person feels highly motivated to do absolutely nothing. If you live to ride motivational highs, you may also ride motivational lows.

Maybe you've experienced the 3 AM motivational wave to change your life (when it's conveniently inconvenient to actually do that). Motivation is feral. Those who try to control it will lose. Those who train to operate in spite of its swings will win.

We train for the habit of moving. The habit of exercising daily. *This ends up becoming the habit of acting against motivational lows when necessary.*

Motivation can and should be utilized when in our favor, but we are never to succumb to its tide over our chosen path. That was the old us. Real power is not exercising for an hour because you're excited about your goal. Real power is having a lousy workout on a day that 99% of people would have chosen to do nothing instead.

Now, I'm not advocating for anyone to overtrain or push themselves beyond healthy limits. I'm advocating for the power of choice when you know you can benefit and become stronger habitually and physically, but have a mental block, negative emotions, and a level of resistance that makes action difficult.

Case in point, I also advocate for allowing yourself to do *less* sometimes. Let's talk about that tomorrow.

Day 48

Allow Yourself to Do Less

"Once we accept our limits, we go beyond them."

~ Albert Einstein

To accept a limit is not weakness, it is a crucial strategic observation that allows us to overcome it. We cannot change our brains quickly (limit), and so we change it slowly but powerfully.

Reader Spotlight: "I loved the one push-up idea. It made so much sense to me. I have what I call a 5x10. Five exercises x 10 reps, with a minimum of one rep. Some days I get all 50 reps and then some. Other days it's just the one."

I've gone through the process I teach in this book, and now I'm years down the mini-habit-into-full-habit road. One core lesson that has stuck with me and allowed me to be consistent is the idea that it's okay to do less.

Once you start working out consistently, you will develop a standard and expected level of intensity. This is overall a good thing, but, when you're at a low point, that high standard might intimidate you; it might convince you to skip a day or two... or three. And that's trouble.

Instead of clinging to soft standards that you have established in these 48 days, it's important to be willing to do less. Doing less is not a sign of weakness; rather, it's a sign of strength to still show up when you're not at your best. That is how you build mental strength!

Doing less than you want is infinitely better than doing nothing at all. Remember that. Give yourself permission to aim lower-- this is your permission to win in any circumstance. And, who knows, once you start moving, it might even energize you to achieve what you originally desired.

I wrote this on a day I lifted weights for half the amount of time I usually do. It was fantastic and much better than nothing. This perspective will keep you consistent and allow you to get better results.

Tomorrow, we discuss the proper order of things when it comes to behavior change. Don't get this one wrong.

Day 49

Integrate, then Optimize

"Everybody is interested in success, but nobody cares about the process behind it."

~ Pratik Gandhi

For something this easy? You always have the time. You always have the energy.

Reader Spotlight: "I thought my goal was stupid easy at just two minutes daily. Kept reading and realized I had to go "stupider & simpler." Now my goal is to put tennis shoes on in the AM period. I don't take them off till I get at least two minutes daily. And BAM! I have not missed a day in seven weeks!"

Have you ever met someone *too friendly*? Even if they have pure intentions, someone who comes on too strong can activate your defenses. But why is this?

Trust and familiarity must come before intimacy.

The same rule goes for your behavior. (Throw the Ab Destroyer 9000 program in storage until you're truly ready for it.) Your current habitual framework (i.e., your brain) needs to befriend a behavior slowly before it will let its guard down and accept the behavior as an important part of life.

Typical exercise programs seem more meaningful at first, but it's like someone trying to kiss you before introducing themselves. Kisses mean more than handshakes, but an unwelcome handshake won't end in a slap. The casual nature of these 60 days is by design. We're building trust and familiarity first.

After you've built familiarity and trust, you can optimize your workouts for the specific results you want. Your mini habit integration phase is creating a deeper biological understanding of why exercise matters and takes it from a means to an end (fragile) to a preference (resilient). Without integration, there's no foundation for behavioral longevity.

Tomorrow's topic sounds strange and possibly too obvious, but it's a powerful mental weapon that you can use inside and outside of this strategy.

Day 50

Why We Should Try

"You may be disappointed if you fail, but you are doomed if you don't try."

~ Beverly Sills

We're so far in now that I want you to reflect on Day 1. How have you changed since then? Try your best each day, and your best will keep getting better.

One of the most valuable lessons I've learned through more than a decade of practicing mini habits is this:

It's very easy not to try, but it isn't much harder to try.

The easiest path is tempting, but once you realize the superior path *can also be made easy*, you will achieve more than you ever have before. We get turned off to the idea of exercise when we inflate it to mean more than it really means. Any movement is exercise. Duration and intensity are variables that we can adjust based on our unique situation each day.

Those who believe that effort must be enormous to count are the ones who are least likely to put forth *any effort at all*. We must be diligent to avoid this mindset with exercise because it opens the door to complete inactivity, which is the worst possible outcome. I'm not sure everyone realizes just *how much better* 10 seconds of jumping around is than doing nothing.

Tomorrow, we enter the home stretch, the final 10 days of this challenge. I call it "A New You." We'll talk about next steps and how to nurture your new habit. And we're starting with steroids, because it's better to know all about them than to know only the upsides or only the downsides.

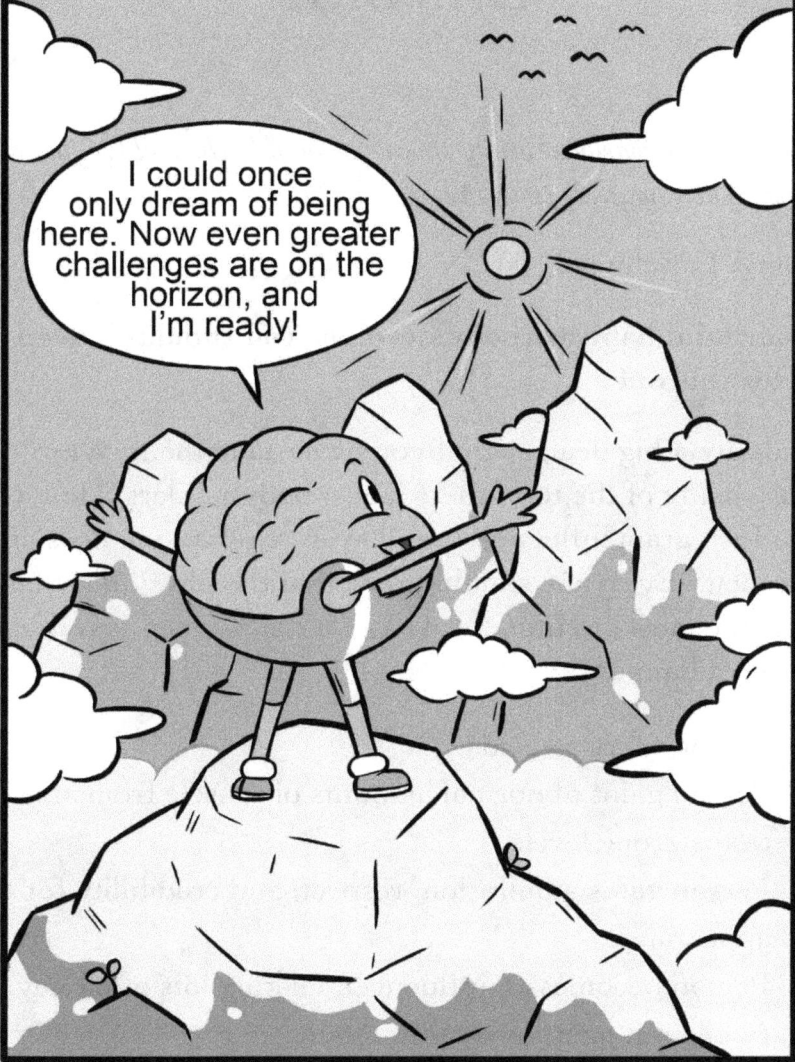

Day 51

Steroids

"An 11-year observational study showed a roughly threefold higher risk for death in steroid users than in nonusers."

~ Thomas L. Schwenk, MD

Do your mini habit without steroids. You shouldn't need them for this one.

Steroids are a big deal, even if you never take them. Why? Because many of the top fitness icons, bodybuilders, Hollywood actors, Instagram influencers, and even regular gym bros are taking them. Everyone should know that the physiques that wow us the most are unnatural. And it's sick when you think about what happens:

1. Person takes steroids.
2. Person gains abnormal amounts of muscle from abnormal testosterone levels.
3. Person gains admiration, respect, and credibility for their appearance.
4. Person becomes an influencer, making lots of money (while not mentioning steroids).
5. Viewers mistakenly think they can follow this person's advice to look like them (when the only possible way is steroids).

A few years ago, I remember watching some videos of an actor talking about his gym routine and diet. I watched, thinking I might find some part of the secret to his success. The secret wasn't mentioned in the video (steroids). They talk about eating broccoli and chicken, while also injecting synthetic testosterone? Transparency about steroid use is important because otherwise it creates unrealistic standards.

What about all the steroid users who say it doesn't take away from their hard work in the gym? Actually, it does, because the hormonal boost is so powerful it overshadows gym work.

A study found that taking steroids *without working out* produced greater gains in size and strength than working out without steroids.[1] That's right, taking steroids and *doing nothing* builds more muscle than working out. It's like magic, but, as the saying goes, nothing is free.

Testosterone is regulated in many places and banned in others because it's dangerous. If there were no downsides to steroids, we'd all be taking them. Why not? To gain so much muscle and strength so easily would be marvelous! Alas, the downsides are downright terrifying.

Before I list a few of the side effects, did you know that steroids can be addictive? That's another serious concern. Now, in the footnote you can see a list of the reasons why steroids are a bad idea, according to the National Health Service in the UK.[2]

In men, steroids can cause breast development, infertility, erectile dysfunction, and a lot more. You had me (scared) at breast development. When men begin taking testosterone, their testes stop producing (as much) testosterone, meaning that, once you start, if you stop, you will be miserable with low testosterone. You can very quickly become dependent on it.

In women, anabolic steroids can cause facial hair growth and body hair, loss of breasts, and... do I need to keep going here?

They can also cause hair loss and acne.

Worst of all, that's the *minor stuff*. Men and women risk heart attack or stroke, liver or kidney failure, and high blood pressure (hypertension). Plus, there are psychological effects. It's a scary and long list, and that's because it's an unnatural amount of an important hormone.

Steroids throw the body out of balance.

Unless you have top 0.00001% genetics, you will never look like steroid users. And steroid users are the ones who get the most attention. This is so important to know as a natural person who exercises, because you can't expect your results to be anywhere near that of a steroid user. Don't let that discourage you; let it encourage you, as your results from exercise are likely better than they seem.

I know I've been frustrated at times when I feel my progress in the mirror doesn't match my effort. But that's when it's helpful to remember that exercise is not *merely* a tool to look better. It's the best way to improve your health, mood, confidence, and energy. It's worth it for those benefits alone. Goodhart's Law warns us against steroids, which sacrifice your health and more in order to increase one measure--your physical strength.

Oh, and if nothing above convinced you, maybe the threat of early death will. Today's leading quote was about a 2024 study which found that steroid users were 2.8 times more likely to die prematurely than nonusers.[3] We've seen so many revered bodybuilders die before the age of 50 due to heart failure. In 2021, 80% of the 15 top professional and high-ranking amateur bodybuilders who died were under age 50.[4]

Steroids aren't worth it. If they were, I would be the first person in line to take them. Keep your mini habit going, and you'll get stronger without risking your health and life.

Tomorrow, we'll discuss exercise obsession. Some people have it. But is it needed to get in great shape?

Day 52

You Don't Need Obsession

"All you need is the plan, the road map, and the courage to press on to your destination."

~ Earl Nightingale

Are you bored with this? If so, that's okay. Real habits are often boring things that you do all the time.

Some people's lives revolve around exercise. As far as hobbies and passions go, it's a healthy one to have. But there's no need for everyone to become obsessed with fitness.

In all areas of life, a person may see another person's extreme lifestyle, and it puts them off the whole idea because they've seen the extreme version. You might look at someone who goes to the gym every day for several hours, for example, and decide that you don't *ever* want to go to the gym. That's an understandable misunderstanding.

Exercise is for everyone in small amounts, for most in moderate amounts, and for far fewer in extreme amounts.

Some people get a powerful and addictive high from exercising or need it for their career as an athlete, actor, or bodybuilder. For the rest of us, you can simply dedicate a few minutes a day to exercise and not think about it otherwise. That can add great value to your health and quality of life.

If you don't want to be a "gym rat," you can think of exercise as a snack--something small and good that you enjoy and occasionally crave. That is a fantastic place to be psychologically.

"I think I'll grab a snack."

"I think I'll walk for 10 minutes on the treadmill."

Easy. Beneficial. Satisfying. ← Can I trademark this?

Snacks taste good and give us energy. We see the benefit there. But a treadmill walk has even better short-term benefits: It will increase our blood flow, improving our brain function and digestion. We'll sleep a bit better that night, too.

Enjoy your exercise-snack today!

Tomorrow, I have a thought-provoking question for you.

Day 53

Exercise <--> Feel Good

"Success doesn't demand a price. Every step forward pays a dividend."

~ David Joseph Schwartz

Every day matters. Remember the goal: it isn't to do 60 days and be done. It's to continue to reshape the relationship. Feel the difference when you move versus not. Internalize the benefits.

Reader Spotlight: "My mini habit would, at least initially, consist of running in place in our backyard if the weather was good or in our laundry room if it wasn't. It felt absurd, like it would accomplish nothing, but it was an exercise commitment that flew under the radar of every excuse that my brain could come up with. My brain simply said, "Sure, whatever, Carl Lewis. Have fun with your 'exercise'. Maybe you'll qualify for the New York City marathon over in the laundry room. [...] Slowly, over several months, exercising has once again become a part of my identity."

There is a great misconception about exercise. It's not something you hear, but it's a common way people think. I know this because I've made this mistake countless times in my life. Most people have. And once you hear the truth, it can really help you overcome resistance to exercise.

The misconception: When I feel good and energized, that's when I'll exercise. This idea seems logical because exercise requires a lot of energy. This thinking causes people to wait or rest instead of exercising.

The truth: The best *reason* to exercise is to feel good and energized. In other words, feeling good is the result, not the prerequisite. If you haven't been exercising, you're not likely to feel good or energized, and so waiting for that feeling will ensure you stay inactive. The exercise is the medicine. It's how you get into that energized state more often.

This is the same issue we run into with motivation. Many think motivation precedes action, when actually, **action is the best motivator** for additional action. Likewise, energy is the result of exercising, not the requirement.

Certainly, there are caveats to this. If you are deeply fatigued, an intense workout might not be a good idea. Still, our focus is on easy mini habits, which are safe and effective in any state. You'll be able to see the energizing effect of even a small amount of activity.

Tomorrow, we'll talk about the habit spectrum. I'll see you then!

Day 54

Habit Spectrum

"Be extra wary of sudden success and attention--they are not built on anything that lasts and they have an addictive pull. And the fall is always painful."

~ Robert Greene

You're stronger, physically and mentally. Today builds on that further.

So... are you there yet? Is your habit established?

While it may be possible to say "yes" to that, please don't view your journey in this way. Let's be careful not to think in binary "yes/no" terms when it comes to habits. A 2009 journal study on habit formation found that habits were formed in an average of 66 days, but with a range of 18 to 254 days![1] Since our habits are mini, they are likely closer to the lower end of that spectrum (18 days), but we want our fitness habit to be *unquestionably strong* and evolve into something greater.

Remember the goal. It isn't to reach Day 60. It's to continually strengthen this habit until it becomes truly unassailable.

Look at habits as a spectrum of behavioral strength, not as an on/off switch.

One habit might be nearly unbreakable while another is hanging on by a thread. You can label them both habits, but that isn't what matters.

"Habit" is a broad label. Our actual concern is about the behavior's strength and role in your life, and whether it's expanding or shrinking.

How many days does it take to form a habit? The question is heavily flawed, because habits are valued by their strength, rather than their existence. You'll know you "get it" when you start celebrating each individual iteration that makes your habit stronger, instead of wondering "when it will happen."

You're at 54 days. Keep your streak alive! The big picture takes care of itself when you focus on mastering how you live each individual day.

Drivers of Exercise Enjoyment
- Early days: increased familiarity
- Later days: long-term benefits, improved performance, and health incentives

Your subconscious always prefers familiar behaviors. That's why, in these early days, we're just getting familiar with exercising daily. You've increased your familiarity with daily exercise without the baggage of societal pressures or extreme workouts souring the deal.

Have you felt better since starting this book? I sure hope so, but as a reminder, this is just the beginning. Think of this method like a slow cooker--it takes longer than nuking food in the microwave, but the end results are *higher quality*.

Alas, I know that everyone wants those big results--increased fitness, weight loss, improved endurance. On Day 32, we talked about *how* small habits become big habits. Tomorrow, we'll talk about *when* you can expect that to happen.

Day 55

How Long Will My Habit Be Embarrassingly Small?

"How long will my habit be embarrassingly small?"

~ You, the Reader

Most fitness programs ask you to be at 100 every day. Real progress is messy and not a straight line. Embrace the ups and downs as long as the overall trend is UP.

Reader Spotlight: "I lost 150 pounds doing just this and have kept it off for close to 10 years."

That's a great question from you. But it's the wrong focus. Everyone wants results, of course, but fast results are often the worst results. Considering how our minds and bodies work, nobody would actually want instant results. That all but guarantees that the changes won't last.

Consider the difference between an **outward result** and an **inward change**. An outward result is almost meaningless if it is soon to be reversed, right? Crash diets, brutal fitness programs, and liposuction are all examples of forced external change. And they all have a strong track record of reverting back to where you started.

A genuine inward change of your brain's preferences is an

engine that can drive outward results for the rest of your life.

We've focused on changing what exercise means to you, and how difficult you find it to be. This change, if we're successful, is going to drive greater raw results *without any extra mental effort.* After Day 60, I will ask you to retake the exercise relationship quiz, and advise you on where to go from there.

The bottom line: Before you concern yourself with ceilings, **you had better have a powerful floor in place.** If exercise isn't something you *know* that you'll do every day, you're not ready to think about ceilings yet. Professional athletes can worry about their physical ceiling because they have already mastered the mental and habitual side of fitness.

Forget ceilings. Chase mastery and consistency first. When you have that floor of "I know I'll do at least a little bit," you can then look to build that into "I know I'll do at least a moderate amount." It's tempting to skip ahead, but patient consistency will yield the best long-term results.

Timing of advancement is difficult to predict. I set this book at 60 days because that's enough to give you a foundation for exercising daily. At the end of the book, I will give you guidance for the days ahead, but to give exact timelines would not be accurate for everyone. We all started from different places and are living in different situations.

What I can tell you is that you should look to continue to build from the floor up, not grasp at ceiling outcomes. **This isn't to say you can't experiment.** If you think you might be ready to jump to full and consistent gym workouts, please try it! You'll find out if you really have that foundation or if you need more time to train at home.

If you take a leap and find out it's too much, don't throw everything away. Don't forget this experience in which you showed perfect or near-perfect consistency for two months. You can modify your mini habit to whatever your current level is or becomes. If it's a year down the road and you're great at working out for at least 20 minutes a day, but your attempt to do full-hour workouts at the gym failed, you don't have to go back to one-minute mini habits. Simply revisit your established floor of 20 minutes, or whatever that may be.

When you increase your exercise expectations, look out for red and green flags.

Red flags (not ready for this level):
- You feel resistance.
- It takes a lot of effort just to get yourself started or to the gym.
- You miss days.
- You're not enjoying it or feel a sense of dread when it's time to exercise.
- It feels like an obligation more than exploration.

Green flags (good to go!):
- You look forward to it.
- You think more about the endorphins and sense of satisfaction you'll get than the work.
- You hate to miss days and rarely do.
- It feels exciting to unlock new levels of strength and fitness.

Note: It may start out as green flags and turn to red flags. This is a sign that you weren't actually ready for it and may have been riding a motivational high. If the green flags last for two months, you should be in the clear and can continue building higher! But remember that no habit is invincible.

On that note, tomorrow we'll discuss what it means to take care of your habit.

Day 56

Take Care of Your Habit

"Even the finest sword plunged into salt water will eventually rust."

~ Sun Tzu

You and your fitness habit must take care of each other. Your part is showing up each day.

We've been framing this behavior as a relationship because it helps us think about it in a healthier way. No more fitness one-night stands! We want to benefit from this for life.

Marital vows tend to include the line "in sickness and in health." It's a promise to take care of the other person as best we can, even if things get difficult. When it comes to a behavior like exercise, things can and will get difficult, and we need the same type of commitment.

Illness may force you to take time off from working out. Will you be eager to come back when you're truly ready, or delay without reason?

Injury may prevent you from exercising at all (or certain body parts). Will you work out in alternate ways? I went to the gym on a cruise ship and saw a woman working out her upper body with a full leg cast on. That was inspiring to see. I don't know about you, but seeing that crushed some of the excuses I've had in the past to skip a workout.

Bouncing back is an important skill, given life's challenges. But it isn't merely resilience; *it's adaptation*. You may find yourself in an airport all day. You may not have access to your regular equipment. Find a way to win the day!

I find I can adapt better when I take a positive and fun approach.

Mindset: Think "fun challenge" over "dreadful effort."
Choice: Choose enjoyable movements and exercises over hated ones.
Location: Work out at home, at the gym, or outside (wherever you enjoy it most).
Accessories: Get a quality water bottle, comfortable workout clothes, and a delicious protein shake recipe.

There's so much you can do to make exercise not only pleasant but something to really look forward to. Feeling great with endorphins flowing afterward is the cherry on top!

This is the same idea as choosing to look at the positive attributes of your partner instead of their flaws. **Nobody's perfect, no body is perfect, and no workout is perfect.** We will have every kind of mental and physical challenge get in the way of frictionless exercise, but that doesn't have to take away from our enjoyment of it.

The best workouts are the ones you didn't feel like doing and did anyway. And they're the most valuable, because they reinforce that it's always a **good decision** to move your body and invest in your health.

In conclusion, to take care of your habit, adapt to difficult circumstances, cultivate positivity and fun, and accept imperfect outcomes. You can count on destructive waves coming for your habit. Your response: Surf's up!

Tomorrow, we talk about the folly of comparison.

Day 57

No Need to Compare

"Your vision will become clear only when you can look into your own heart. Who looks outside, dreams; who looks inside, awakes."

~ Carl Jung

Do your mini habit today. Go on. I'll wait here until you're done.

Alright, let me ask you a question. Are you the strongest man or woman in the world? Are you the fastest? Are you the fittest? If you answered no, then the following applies to you.

It is arbitrary and worthless to compare yourself to any other person.

With the exception of the literal strongest person, *everyone is behind. Everyone.* But being behind someone else's fitness level is not a problem, nor is it relevant. If you are exercising to be like or look like someone else, or perhaps what you deem "normal," let me introduce you to a better and more powerful motive.

Exercise for yourself. For your health. For your lifestyle and well-being. Even for your own vanity. External motivators are always weaker and less motivating than doing something for yourself. They may appear stronger at first, but in the process of increasing your fitness level, nothing can beat the allure of becoming a better version of *you.*

There will always be someone stronger or fitter, and that's completely okay, because, unless you are in a bodybuilding competition, well, this isn't a competition!

I'll never forget the day. I looked over and saw a kid, maybe 17 years old, benching over 300 pounds easily. There I was, older and considerably weaker. Bummer. But it turns out that you don't need to bench 300 pounds to be healthy, have energy, be confident, and feel amazing.

When you see someone else in the gym or in a public place who is further along, it may help to remember that *they* are behind others. Also, the most impressive-looking people use steroids (which are not worth the health consequences).

If someone else makes you feel inadequate in any way, remind yourself that they (external source) cannot determine the standard for you. You create your own standard, and it starts with where you are right now. And pay very close attention to the next sentence.

Your standard right now should be *lower* than it will be later.

Most exercise literature will try to "pump you up" by telling you to demand a higher standard for yourself. They are asking you to shoot yourself in the foot. You will get fitter and stronger by *accepting where you are right now*. Don't pretend that you're a world-class athlete or bodybuilder if you're not. Don't think you have to act like one either.

"But Stephen, I feel so far behind and have so much work to do!"

Behind what? You are exactly where you are. If you desire to improve to a much higher level, that's fine, but bear in mind that desire isn't the mechanism of change.

Change only happens when you live your day differently

than before and do it repeatedly.

Life is made of days, not weeks or months. This isn't a two-month program, it's a 60-day program, designed to change how you perceive exercise within the context of a single day. If you can make exercise a regular and enjoyable part of your day, you win. After that, it's simply a matter of leveraging that habit to reach your ideal level of fitness.

If you try to "go for it" before you have that base, you'll fall off. We've all done it. I've done extreme workout programs and even saw nice visible progress in 20 days. Not only did I quit, but I stopped working out as much afterward. Because I felt like I had to do these extremely draining workouts, and my brain (let alone my body) wasn't close to ready for that level. So the net result of that program was *less exercise*.

This is the problem we're going to correct. Let's get to know exercise at a level that's comfortable and nonthreatening. Exercise is valuable in small doses. Throughout the whole process, we're constantly building momentum instead of losing it (as in extreme workout programs that drain you).

As you increase your capabilities, your standards will <u>naturally and automatically</u> increase too. Think about this! We don't want to outstrip our capabilities because we have made an unrealistic standard. We want to build ourselves up to a point where higher standards are realistic and natural.

Tomorrow, we talk about working out when sick and the one guy who famously did it.

Day 58

Working out with Pneumonia

"I can't die, it would ruin my image."

~ Jack LaLanne

Do your mini habit today unless you have pneumonia.

Jack LaLanne was one of the most famous fitness icons in recent memory. Unfortunately, he was mortal like the rest of us, but he lived to an impressive 96 years old. What he did the day before his death is even more remarkable than his long lifespan.

LaLanne had developed a routine of working out for two hours every day. He would work out with weights for 90 minutes and swim for 30 minutes. And when I say he didn't miss days, *he didn't miss days*. The day before he died from pneumonia, he still completed his two-hour workout. How that's even possible is beyond me.

Now, I wouldn't advocate for any 96-year-old with pneumonia to attempt to work out, but the fact that he did shows the relationship he had developed with exercise. He absolutely loved it. It was integral to who he was.

While you or I may never reach LaLanne-levels of love and dedication to fitness, we can certainly reach heights that would shock our closest friends and family.

Many people today have time to exercise, enough energy to

exercise, and even exercise equipment in their own homes and *still* choose not to exercise regularly. I'm not shaming anyone. I'm saying that it's all about the relationship. Jack LaLanne fought in his dying days to exercise against all odds (96 with pneumonia) because of the relationship he had with it.

LaLanne is a fascinating case study. He was a sickly child, a self-described "sugarholic," with many health problems. He described this time as "hell on earth." When he joined the YMCA and started working out, he said it saved his life.[1] If something saves your life, you're going to love it!

I don't know the exact trajectory of LaLanne's relational transformation with exercise, but I know it was more extreme and intense than most cases. I believe that was in large part due to his young age. It's easier to build new behaviors when you're young because they're competing with fewer and less-established behaviors than someone who is older.

Exercise is powerful enough to completely transform a person's mind, health, and life, and I hope you've experienced a taste of that power in this journey. These benefits will continue to build as you strengthen the habit and your body.

Tomorrow, we debate the age-old question--quantity or quality?

Day 59

Quantity vs Quality

"The reason I exercise is for the quality of life I enjoy."

~ Kenneth H. Cooper (age 93)

Our journey is almost at an end. But for you, it has just begun.

Reader Spotlight: "It's been years now, and I haven't missed a day of doing my habits. That's because the requirement is so small, and I have kept it small. Most days I do more, but on the days I am overwhelmed or ill, I just do the mini amount."

Some think that people exercise for a longer life (quantity), but I find the greater benefit is quality of life. Your body feels and functions much better when you use it.

Fitness in particular seems to garner incorrect assumptions about what makes it so great. I can demonstrate this with a simple observation.

When someone is in peak physical condition, almost everyone sees their appearance as *the* big benefit. "Wow, (s)he looks amazing." I used to think that too, but now I think, "Wow, (s)he must feel amazing." All else equal, a fit body has far fewer aches, pains, and health problems than an unfit body. It has better protection against disease.

Health benefits from exercise are the most addictive. Once you feel the difference between sedentary living and active living *and* have built an active habit to support the lifestyle, it's truly difficult to go back. It simply feels too good to quit.

Since these are mini habits, and we have been focused on the relationship more than the raw numbers, you have only scratched the surface of how good it can feel to exercise. I will never forget that when I first started my one push-up per day, I felt better and stronger even from that.

Because of genetics and dietary choices, not everyone is going to look like a fitness model when they train hard. But we can all feel significantly better by being active. Beauty fades with time anyway, but you can continue to feel good into old age if you continue to move.

It's funny: I'm on a cruise ship as I write this. Unprompted, an elderly gentleman on the ship told me today, "The key to life is to keep moving." Needless to say, I heartily agreed!

Tomorrow is the last day. See you there!

Day 60

The Last and Most Important Lesson

"Seventy percent of success is showing up.

Eighty percent of success is showing up.

Ninety percent of success is showing up."

~ Woody Allen

I'm quite certain that Woody Allen said at least one of these three quotes. But I'm not certain which percentage was the actual quote, and I'm also not sure he didn't say more than one of these. So I've included all three options and you can pick your favorite one. Thankfully, the meaning is the same. The large majority of success comes from showing up!

To seal a profound accomplishment of exercising every single day for 60 days in a row, do your mini habit today. And then give yourself a big round of applause, or dance, or do some other kind of celebratory action.

Our final discussion is a critical reminder of the two stages of any action.

The first stage is **before action**. This is where you deliberate between multiple options: Do the dishes? Watch TV? Exercise? Go bowling? It can last a short time or a long time.

The second stage is **in action**. You're in motion at this point, and the focus shifts from what to do to how to do it.

Your number one goal and priority for exercise should always be to reach the second stage as quickly as possible. Get in motion. Once you're there, you can figure out the rest. Why? Because once in motion, you've already won.

Think about yourself in the past or anyone you know who has struggled to exercise. Which of the following has been the issue?

1. They don't work out.
2. Their workouts aren't good enough.

If someone is struggling, the problem is 99.99% of the time going to be #1. They don't *attempt* to exercise enough. In other words, they get stuck in stage one. They may think about exercise and overthink it, but rarely do they act.

In these 60 days, you've seen what happens when you act. It isn't always amazing, but it does always create real and meaningful progress. And cumulatively, those daily wins build upon each other. You get stronger and faster, mentally and physically. Your confidence increases each day you succeed. You start to see exercise in its purest form, away from the baggage and expectations.

This is the way to improve your fitness and your life. Nothing can stop you if you know how to thrust yourself into action. Leave behind the days in which you deliberate over what to do and how much of it is "good enough" to matter. Now you know that every little bit counts. Now you know that when you consistently seek out small wins, they accumulate into bigger wins.

Before the concluding chapter, I have one last suggestion for the future. Try not to box in this idea to the construct of "once a day." That is the standard mini habit and it works well, but this concept needn't be limited by that. There are hundreds or thousands of small pockets of time within each day to move a little bit more than you would have.

The simple, obvious daily application of this is taking the stairs or parking far away. I take the stairs frequently, and I'm usually the *only person* taking them. The modern world has seemingly decided to avoid this small amount of exercise at all costs. The same people who wonder why they can't get themselves to work out more are avoiding this free, easy, and fast opportunity to activate their bodies. If you don't take the stairs, you've decided that it's better to move less.

I have a pull-up bar in one of my doorways. Any time I walk by, I can pump out a pull-up or three. Or I can hang from it to stretch my arms and back. Anywhere there's ground is an opportunity to do push-ups. If you look, there are countless opportunities to take small wins. And I promise you, if you pay attention to these and seek them out, their cumulative effect will shock you.

You've built a foundation to last in these 60 days. I sincerely hope you love to exercise now or at least tolerate it more than you used to. Now go out into the world, move more, and enjoy it.

Read on for the conclusion and next steps in your journey.

Part III

Conclusion

The Battle and the War

You've won the first 60 mini-battles and the first big battle. Sixty straight days of exercise is extraordinary. But you might be wondering when you'll win the war.

The truth? The war never ends, but you can effectively win it for the rest of your life by continuing to nurture this new way of living. Habits can always get stronger or weaker, meaning we aren't looking for a destination so much as *mastering the process of strengthening the habit*. First, you master the process. Then, the process teaches you to love the behavior and, at that point, winning every day becomes second nature.

In these early days, it helps to track your behavior. It brings accountability and reinforces your decision. There's a small reward of satisfaction when you "check" or "X" another day. When the behavior is a habit, though, tracking becomes an unnecessary chore. You don't need to track what will definitely happen!

These days, I don't track my exercise. I enjoy exercising daily and I do track my workout metrics for strength and hypertrophy purposes, but more intense exercise sometimes requires rest, and I just listen to my body. When you have complete confidence that you'll show up even without tracking your workouts, you know you've developed a strong habit.

That being said, many people enjoy tracking and planning their exercise long after it has become an established habit. I'm a spontaneous person and so I only track behaviors before a habit is established. Do whatever works best for you!

What's Next?

Now it's time to revisit your relationship with exercise to see if it has improved in these 60 days. Answer as honestly as possible!

Take the post-book quiz now to see how you've changed: minihabits.com/exercise-quiz-after/

What did you score on your post-book exercise assessment?

Level 1 (0-20): Strong aversion
Level 2 (21-40): Some discomfort
Level 3 (41-60): Neutral
Level 4 (61-80): Positive feelings
Level 5 (81-100): Love/Addiction

Recommended Options Based on Your New Score

I'm going to recommend some next steps based on what you scored. But of course, you can do whatever you want. If an option sounds right for you even though it's under a different level than the one you scored, feel free to choose it.

Levels 1-2

The goal of this book was to increase you two levels over this 60 days. So, if you started at level 1 (strong dislike), we wanted you to get to level 3 (neutral). If you're still at level 1 and went through all 60 days successfully, I'd be surprised.

If you're still at level 1 or 2 but you found this experience tolerable or even enjoyable, why not give it another round? You may need more time to adjust and that's perfectly fine. Remember that progress is *not* linear inside the brain. That means that sometimes the results seem to happen on Day 73 all at once. It also means that scoring the same on the assessment on Day 60 as Day 1, while not ideal, is not necessarily a total failure. For example, you might have a higher raw score but still be in the same category. That's a small win, and if this book teaches anything, it's that small wins are valuable.

If you managed to level up from level 1 to 2, that's a *massive* win. You moved the scale! A small positive move in the relationship can produce exponentially better exercise consistency and experiences.

Recommendations:

1. Start this book over at Day 1 and go another 60 days. Reinforce these critical ideas and build an even stronger habit.

2. Continue doing your mini habit without the book's guidance. You know the drill by now. I'd recommend that you continue to track it until it feels completely pointless (when you have absolutely zero doubts about doing your behavior). Or until you reach level 3, which is neutrality towards exercise.

Levels 2-3

At this level, you're close to the tipping point or right at it. As your guide, this tempts me to introduce you to the next level, but that's quickly overridden by the importance of improving the relationship to a stable place first. The tricky thing about exercise is that the best and most beneficial version of it (intense) is the most repulsive when you don't like it (it's also the most addictive kind when you like exercise).

I have always been a "I hate mushrooms" guy. The taste, the texture, no thanks. But I once had a homemade dish in Germany with mushrooms in it and really liked it, even the mushrooms! The mushrooms were not overly strong or the main part of the dish. Rather, they were a supporting piece of a really delicious meal. This experience opened my mind to eating mushrooms in general and I don't hate them nearly as much as I used to.

Lesson: When someone dislikes something, barraging them with the most extreme versions of it is not likely to win their favor! Subtle exposure, however, especially in a favorable context, can move the needle.

Therefore, at this level, be wary of suddenly going nuts with intense exercise. If you have any lingering distaste for exercise, extreme exercise is most likely going to heighten that distaste, just like being forced to eat a massive mushroom could move mushrooms right back to my do-not-eat list.

Recommendations:

1. Spice things up with a progression system. This is more than a mini habit, but it keeps things manageable. Example: Increase your mini habit floor from one push-up to ten. Or do rolling increases on a weekly basis (at the start of each week, add one more minimum rep). Try to keep it easy enough that you won't fail to hit it even on your worst day(s). This can make it more interesting while keeping you on track to further improve the relationship.

2. Evolve your mini habit into an elastic habit (another book of mine). An elastic habit has three levels of success (mini, plus, elite). Upside targets can inject more variety and excitement into the behavior and tracking. Since it's completely optional to do the upper level, it won't make you feel like you're being pushed too hard. You can always just do the mini level.

Levels 3-5

The purpose of your mini habit journey was to improve your relationship with exercise. If you're at this level, that means you're at least neutral and probably find some enjoyment in exercise.

Fantastic. You have the single best foundation for any behavior: if you tolerate it, like it, or love it, you can go far with it.

With a neutral-to-positive relationship with exercise, the natural next step is to increase the intensity and duration of your workouts, but in a smart way. If you want to take things to the next level, here's what I recommend.

Recommendations:

I think the optimal end goal for most is to get a gym membership. Strength training is great for men and women. Gyms often have sports courts, and group fitness classes are fun. I say this as someone who has a garage gym in my home. While I have a great setup at home to work out, I still prefer the gym for these reasons.

1. I get out of the house. I work from home, so maybe this is more for me than most people. It's a healthy escape. The gym may become your sanctuary and a place to regain sanity in this crazy world.

2. The equipment at gyms is comprehensive and high quality. Many of my favorite exercises aren't possible in my home gym, and my equipment isn't as nice.

3. The drive to go to the gym makes it easy to commit to a workout, even if I don't feel it that day. Pro tip: Before a workout, you may or may not feel "up to it," but you will never regret doing it. It always feels great afterwards! I've experienced this hundreds of times in my life, but it takes a long time to internalize it, so be patient with yourself. Your home gym is convenient, but it means there are a lot more distractions around. At the gym, you have one purpose; it's clear and you leave when you're done.

4. I treat myself to a takeout meal afterwards. It's part of what makes the routine so fun for me. My gym, like many, is in a shopping center, so it's convenient. If something like this can sweeten your gym routine, do it. It can be the boost you need.

But, hold on a second. After completing your 60 days of mini habits, you might not be totally ready to jump into a gym routine headfirst. I know, because I've been there! If you're at a neutral, level 3 exercise relationship, a demanding gym commitment and extreme expectations can quickly send you to Couchville.

There's a way to ease into it.

One of my favorite mini habits is to put on gym clothes. That's the first step you take when you go to the gym, right? Try it and watch in awe as you find yourself walking to the car and driving away to pump iron or get on the stair master. I've heard *countless* stories of this working wonders, including people saying, "I just made a mini habit to put on my running shoes, and in X months I was running for miles every day."

If you're not into that idea, you can use my favorite one--**just show up at the gym**. Do whatever you want when you get there. Play around. Go intense. Whatever you want. If you show up, you've won. If you're like me, you'll want to do at least a little bit of working out to make your trip worthwhile. But try your best to limit expectations. If you push yourself too hard too soon and expect that every time, the gym will not look very appealing the next time you consider going.

The best part of this is that you can keep this as your philosophy for the rest of your life. **Just show up.** I LOVE intense exercise now, and my goal to just show up remains unchanged. There's a difference in what "show up" means today as I've leveled up my fitness and habit. That will happen organically.

When I was in a neutral relationship with exercise, I had internalized some of the benefits of exercise but didn't really enjoy the effort required. I'd show up and have decent, low-pressure workouts. It was a positive experience that allowed my brain to adjust and see the enormous benefits. Over time, I grew to absolutely love it.

Let your "show up" expectations grow organically. Don't force any program or system until you're at that level. Look at the gym as a *playground* initially and let yourself do whatever exercise appeals to you at the time.

I understand some people like to be more organized, and, to you folks, go ahead and plan your workout. But please remember to **make the experience as pleasant as possible**. Don't scare yourself away, because this could be the start of a new habit that will transform your life. Especially in the early days, make a rule that you can leave the gym *at any time*. This is important!

As mentioned on Day 41, I track my strength training workouts with the Hevy app for Android and Apple. This is the best one I've found, and it's free. When you love exercising, it's fun and satisfying to beat your best sprint times or your previous bench press, or improve your endurance on the exercise bike. I thought about using an app like this earlier in the process, but I felt a sense of being overwhelmed by it, so I wisely backed off until I *knew I was ready*.

Final Thoughts and My Experience

Exercise is the best and closest human experience to leveling up in a video game. I find that addictive, both in video games and in the gym. The human body is *incredible* at adapting. This is why we get stronger, faster, and fitter with training.

If we're going to be lifting these heavy things all the time, the body says, *we should build more muscle*. When we sit around all day, however, the body has no need to get stronger, and we miss out on life-supercharging benefits.

In my journey, exercise changed from annoying work that I'm supposed to do to something far greater:

- Feeling like a kid again on my bike
- Feeling like a beast after an upper-body workout
- I admit I'm still not loving leg day (better, though)
- The key to feeling great and sleeping like an elephant-tranquilized baby cloud surrounded by cotton angels playing binaural beats on their harps
- A near-panacea for all of my prior aches and pains. I don't get crippling tension headaches anymore. My back went from always hurting to almost never hurting. It's unbelievable to me that my *years* of upper back issues have been silenced by weightlifting.

The lifestyle riches you gain from exercise are astounding. You will continue to unlock them and fall more and more in love with this activity that once seemed like a hassle. It's the *best and most enjoyable* thing you can do. Some people never get the chance to fully feel this, realize this, understand it on a deep level, and love it. But I hope that you continue to build toward this.

That's it. That's the roadmap I recommend after your 60 days of success. The final section of this book is a short sendoff with final tips to help you in your journey.

A Living Book

The purpose of this book was to help you change your

relationship with exercise **first**, and through that foundation, build it into a habit that can scale. Importantly, *neither* of these achievements makes you invincible to regression. Your behavior and brain can always change, for better and for worse, a blessing and a curse. *Narrator: And so began his rap career.*

I call this a living book because it is your active, daily, time-relevant sidekick for 60 days. If you ever need a refresher or feel as if your relationship with exercise has soured again, I invite you to come back and experience these 60 days again with me. Even if you're beyond the mini habit stage, you will benefit from the concepts and can easily adapt your targets to your current level.

Thank you for reading my book. If this helped you, the best way to thank me is to share it with others. On social media, via email, or in person. Most impactful of all, I'd be grateful if you left a review. Reviews are the lifeblood of any book's success.

Finally, I want to say congratulations on completing this challenge. You've built a behavioral foundation for fitness and improved your relationship with exercise. I wish you the best in your fitness journey and in life!

Cheers,

Stephen Guise

Other Books by Stephen Guise

Check out minihabits.com for information on my other books! Here are my other creations.

Mini Habits (Book & Video Course)

My first book! This is the book that started the small habits craze that has taken over the publishing industry in the last decade. It's a worldwide bestseller in 21 languages and people love it. I also made it into a video course, which has over 20,000 students!

Mini Habits for Weight Loss (Book & Video Course)

Diets have been shown to make you gain weight, even more than not dieting. Instead, try this habit-driven approach to weight loss, and your changes can last.

How to Be an Imperfectionist (Book)

This book applies *Mini Habits* to the problem of perfectionism. If you struggle with depression, fear, and inaction, this book has a lot to offer. I receive a lot of emails from readers about this book.

Elastic Habits (Book)

This is *Mini Habits* with a twist! Instead of just having a small daily goal, elastic habits give you the option for mini (easy), plus (medium), and elite (hard) wins every day. Some days are better than others, and an elastic habit can adapt to the unique texture of each day.

The Magic of Momentum (Book)

At the heart of all my books is momentum. *The Magic of Momentum* explores the magic behind small steps and the momentum they create. It will change your perspective. This is my highest rated book!

Questions or inquiries?

Email me: stephen@minihabits.com

References

Important Definitions and Ideas

[1] There's a key difference between addiction to exercise and drug addiction. Exercise requires immense effort, in both the short term (the exercise itself) and the long term (the commitment to make it a habit). Drugs require no effort to begin (just consume it) or get addicted to (instant euphoria brings repeat customers). Drugs would be better than exercise, except that they harm our minds and bodies while exercise makes us happier and stronger, inside and out.

Mini Habits Crash Course

[1] First, I would go to 1986 and put all of my money into the Microsoft IPO. Then I would fast-forward to 1999 and cash out my roughly 66,000% gain. With the proceeds, I would buy the Detroit Lions. In the 2000 NFL draft, I would select Tom Brady with the 181st pick instead of Quinton Reese (sorry Quinton) before the Patriots take him at 199 overall. (My other picks would be good, too.)

Many People Quit Goals around This Time

[1] "What Does Science Say about All the Failed New Year's Resolutions?" CORDIS, 2023. https://cordis.europa.eu/article/id/442773-trending-science-what-does-science-say-about-all-the-failed-new-year-s-resolutions.

[2] R.F. Oman and A.C. King. "Predicting the Adoption and Maintenance of Exercise Participation Using Self-Efficacy and Previous Exercise Participation Rates." *American Journal of Health Promotion* (*AJHP*), 12(3): 154-161. https://pubmed.ncbi.nlm.nih.gov/10176088/

Respect Goodhart's Law

[1] Christopher Mattson, Reamer L Bushardt, and Anthony R Artino. "'When a Measure Becomes a Target, it Ceases to Be a Good Measure.'" *Journal of Graduate Medical Education*, Feb 13, 2021, 13(1): 2-5. https://www.ncbi.nlm.nih.gov/pmc/articles/PMC7901608/

[2] TMZ staff. "Bodybuilder Jodi Vance Dies at 20 after Suffering Heart Attack." TMZ, March 4, 2025. https://www.tmz.com/2025/03/04/bodybuilder-jodi-vance-dead-heart-attack-arnold-sports-festival/

Why Exercise Is a Panacea

[1] John Medina. *Brain Rules: 12 Principles for Surviving and Thriving at Work, Home, and School* (pp. 21-22). Pear Press. Kindle edition.

As Easy as Smoking

[1] Source not found.

Welcome to Non-Linear Progression

[1] S&P 500 returns since 1928. https://www.officialdata.org/us/stocks/s-p-500/1928?amount=100&amp=&endYear=2023

I Can Tell with One Question

[1] E. Stamatakis, M.N. Ahmadi, J.M.R. Gill, C. Thøgersen-Ntoumani, M.J. Gibala, A. Doherty and Mark Hamer. "Association of wearable device-measured vigorous intermittent lifestyle physical activity with mortality." *Nat Med* **28**, 2521-2529 (December 8, 2022). https://doi.org/10.1038/s41591-022-02100-x.

[2] *The New York Times*. "2-minute exercise bursts can have big health benefits." https://www.nytimes.com/2022/12/08/well/move/exercise-bursts-benefits.html.

Sedentary Habits Aren't All Bad

[1] My editor added this nugget of truth: "Remember, all animals sit: dogs sit, lions sit, rabbits sit, birds sit. It's a normal behavior and not at all unhealthy. Only an excess of it is abnormal and unhealthy."

Is Exercise Miserable or Fun?

[1] The song is "The Man" by The Killers, if you're curious. Its length is 4 minutes and 10 seconds, which seems to be the perfect amount of time for four rounds if I'm shooting well and hustling after the ball.

[2] M.M. Atakan, Y. Li, Ş.N. Koşar, H.H. Turnagöl, X. Yan. "Evidence-Based Effects of High-Intensity Interval Training on Exercise Capacity and Health: A Review with Historical Perspective." *Int J Environ Res Public Health*, July 5, 2021,18(13): 7201. doi: 10.3390/ijerph18137201. PMID: 34281138; PMCID: PMC8294064 https://pmc.ncbi.nlm.nih.gov/articles/PMC8294064/#sec5-ijerph-18-07201.

[3] M. Heydari, J. Freund and S.H. Boutcher. "The Effect of High-Intensity Intermittent Exercise on Body Composition of Overweight Young Males." *Journal of Obesity*. doi: 10.1155/2012/480467. Epub 2012 Jun 6. https://pmc.ncbi.nlm.nih.gov/articles/PMC3375095/#sec4

The Best Exercise

[1] J.A. King, L.K. Wasse, D.R. Broom, D.J. Stensel. "Influence of Brisk Walking on Appetite, Energy Intake, and Plasma Acylated Ghrelin." *Medicine and Science in Sports and Exercise,* March 2010, 42(3): 485-492. doi: 10.1249/MSS.0b013e3181ba10c4. https://pubmed.ncbi.nlm.nih.gov/19952806/

Steroids

[1] Shalender Bhasin, Thomas W. Storer, Nancy Berman, Carlos Callegari, Brenda Clevenger, Jeffrey Phillips, Thomas J. Bunnell, Ray Tricker, Aida Shirazi, and Richard Casaburi. "The Effects of Supraphysiologic Doses of Testosterone on Muscle Size and Strength in Normal Men." *New England Journal of Medicine*, July 4, 1996, (335) (1): 1-7. https://doi.org/10.1056/nejm199607043350101.

[2] Physical effects

Effects of anabolic steroids in men can include:

reduced sperm count, infertility, shrunken testicles, erectile dysfunction, hair loss, breast development, increased risk of prostate cancer, severe acne, stomach pain

In women, anabolic steroids can cause:

facial hair growth and body hair, loss of breasts, swelling of the clitoris, a deepened voice, an increased sex drive, problems with periods, hair loss, severe acne

In addition, both men and women who take anabolic steroids can develop any of the following medical conditions:

heart attack or stroke, liver or kidney problems or failure, high blood pressure (hypertension), blood clots, fluid retention, high cholesterol

Psychological effects

Misusing anabolic steroids can also cause the following psychological or emotional effects:

aggressive behaviour, mood swings, paranoia, manic behaviour, hallucinations and delusions

[3] Thomas Schwenk. "Higher Mortality Is Associated with Anabolic Steroid Use." *NEJM*, March 19, 2024. https://www.jwatch.org/na57257/2024/03/19/higher-mortality-associated-with-anabolic-steroid-use.

[4] Guillermo Escalante, Dillon Darrow, V.N. Ambati, Daniel L. Gwartney, and Rick Collins. "Dead Bodybuilders Speaking from the Heart: An Analysis of Autopsy Reports of Bodybuilders That Died Prematurely." *Journal of Functional Morphology and Kinesiology*, Nov 24, 2022, (7)4: 105. https://doi.org/10.3390/jfmk7040105.

Habit Spectrum

[1] P. Lally, C.H.M. van Jaarsveld, H.W.W. Potts and J. Wardle. "How are habits formed: Modelling habit formation in the real world." *Eur. J. Soc. Psychol.*, , July 16, 2009, 40: 998-1009. doi: 10.1002/ejsp.674

Working out with Pneumonia

[1] EMMYTVLEGENDS.ORG. *Jack LaLanne on his poor childhood health*. YouTube video, 5:54. https://www.youtube.com/watch?v=c67x-uymujQ

www.ingramcontent.com/pod-product-compliance
Lightning Source LLC
Chambersburg PA
CBHW062053270326
41931CB00013B/3050